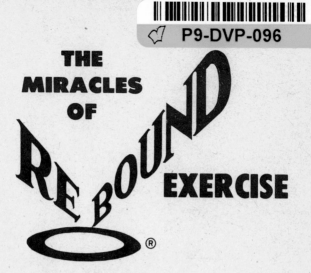

THE MIRACLES OF REBOUND EXERCISE

By Albert E. Carter

For information on the purchase of rebound exercise equipment contact your local Distributor. If none is available contact The National Institute of Reboundology and Health, Inc., and we will forward your request to the appropriate people.

Copyright © 1979

The National Institute of Reboundology & Health, Inc.
7416 212th S.W., Edmonds, WA 98020
Telephone (206) 774-6403 or (800) 426-1333

All Rights Reserved

ISBN 0-938302-01-9

Reprinted 1980
Revised 1980
Reprinted 1981

Printed in U.S.A.

Table of Contents

Introduction

**It looks too
simple . . . it
IS simple!**

That is probably the biggest argument against it. How could anything that simple be so good for you . .

If Rebound Exercise was a little more complicated or caused greater discomfort, it would probably be more popular. But it isn't and doesn't. The fact is, it just happens to be the most effective way to efficiently tap three energy sources simultaneously ... sources that have not previously been considered when we exercise.

Read how thousands[1] of folks each month are discovering this unique method of eliminating bone-jarring, crippling shock to their weight-bearing joints. Eliminating all that, they still get their vitally important aerobic exercise in the convenience, privacy, and safety of their homes.

In a world of torturing, time-consuming exercise programs, this amazing book will shock you with the simplicity of the physical requirements you need to keep in shape.

Learn how easily thousands[2] have overcome aching back problems, eliminated stress, or shed ugly, unhealthy fat.

---

[1] Today, it is estimated that there are over 30 manufacturing companies in the United States selling a combined total of over 20,000 rebound exercise units each month. This has been expanding by approximately 20% a month.

[2] Most people using rebound exercise who have a history of back problems have indicated definite improvement in as little as one or two weeks.

Understand how simple arthritic pains have been eliminated without medication; how other seemingly unsurmountable physical problems have just disappeared.

Find out why Dr. Henry Savage, M.D.[3] says, "Never in my 35 years as a practicing physician have I found any exercise method, at any price, that will do more for the physical body than Rebound Exercise."

Experience Rebound Exercise for yourself. You will agree with Dr. Arland Fuhr, D.C.[4] who states, "I not only feel better when I rebound regularly, but the patients I have involved with Rebound Exercise are recommending it to their friends."

You'll understand why visual therapists have been using Rebound Exercise successfully for over 30 years to improve their patients' vision.[5]

Be aware of this startling new break-through in education that is not merely for the handicapped student. This marvelous concept is available to you.

This text is being written to explain a specific type of exercise. We will analyze the affects of rebound exercise on the human body. Physiologists attempt to explain all aspects of bodily function, including chemical reactions that occur in cells throughout the body, transmission of nerve impulses, movement of the muscles, reproduction, and even such minute details as the transfer formation of light energy into chemical energy to excite the eyes. We will limit our responses only to the G-force loading impact on the body.

The human being is actually automated. We don't have to learn how to function to exist. That we are sensing, feeling, and increasing in knowledge throughout our lives attests that we are automated in spite of our ignorance of ourselves.

[3] 1975 statement by Dr. Henry Savage, M.D., Seattle, Washington.
[4] 1979 statement by Dr. Arland Fuhr, D.C., Redwood Falls, Minn.
[5] See Chapter XII, p.p. 109.

The study of human physiology brings us to astute awareness of the intricate way the body must adjust to its environment to survive; and we stand in awe when we realize that the human body is self-healing and self-adjusting when given proper rest, nutrition, and exercise.

Most physiology studies talk of differences between various systems and organs of the body. This study will present to you similarities that exist. The most revolutionary concepts are usually very simple. The lasting ones are usually true. However, our advanced scientific ego demands that all new ideas must be conceived in a laboratory test tube after years of investigation and extensive study by a team of researchers. The new idea must then be incubated by sophisticated engineers of industry until rendered completely safe and harmless, ready for public consumption. It is then marketed by a conglomerate.

We, as consumers, accept this as part of life. Until a simple truth stands in front of us and slaps us in the face, it seldom gets our attention. We then murmur to ourselves, "That is so true and simple! I wish I had said that!" or, "That's so logical! Why haven't we heard that before?"

Rebound Exercise is one of those simple, logical truths that belong to all of us. Only this time, I said something about it.

Albert E. Carter

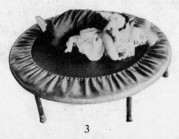

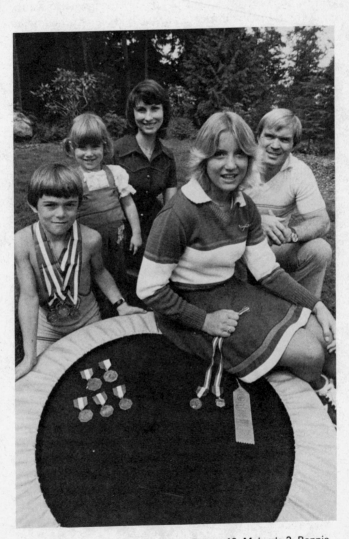

THE CARTER FAMILY: Left to right, Darren 10, Melynda 3, Bonnie, Wendie 14, and Al.

Chapter I
The Often Invisible Obvious

"Darren, listen to me. You only have one more minute to go. The score is 7 to 8. It doesn't make any difference if he beats you by one point or ten. In this next minute, you've got to explode! You're stronger than he is. You have better balance, and your wrestling moves are better, but you've got to want it. He's only one point ahead of you, so you have to throw everything you've ever learned at him. This is it!"

Darren's face was flushed and he was breathing hard, but his eyes flashed with determination as he accepted the challenge. I was on my knees looking at him straight in the face as I had many times before in the last two years. I held his wrists, shaking them slightly to help him relax. It was the last thirty-second rest period in his final match of the year. I heard my voice say the same things I said previously, but this time there was a sense of urgency.

I looked over his shoulder, sized up his opponent again, and reviewed quickly what had happened the first two minutes of this match. Darren's moves were good but too conservative, and I had to admit this was the best kid Darren had faced all year.

The referee signaled the end of the rest period. I said, "Darren, do you want this match?"

"Yes! Yes!" he said with the determination of a winner.

"Then explode! Throw it all at him because you won't have another chance!"

He turned, quickly moved to the center of the mat, crouched and waited for the referee to signal the beginning of the final minute. I could see his 45 pound body quiver with resolve, and I knew that, regardless of the outcome, he would give it everything he had.

The whistle blew and I felt my own body tighten, my muscles automatically moving with Darren's swift attack as he sprang for the double-leg. He went in clean, and the points were awarded quickly. His opponent fought back, but every move met unbeatable quickness, balance and strength.

The next 45 seconds flew by, but they weren't as quick as Darren; three points for a near pin and then an attempted reversal. Darren rolled right on through and ended on top again; and then the towel was thrown in to signal the referee that time had run out.

I felt my body spring into the air, and from someplace in the distance I heard my own voice letting out a war whoop. The wrestlers shook hands, then the referee raised Darren's hand. I staggered out onto the mat, my legs as weak as if I'd fought the match.

"We won! Thanks dad!" he gasped as I picked him up, hugged him, put him on my shoulder, and carried him off the mat to the arms of Bonnie, his mother, and Wendie and Melynda, his sisters.

When all the scores were tallied, Darren was in a three-way tie for first place in the National Kids Wrestling Championships in the 45-pound class, eight years and under. (Since the first publication, he has won the 1979 National Kids Wrestling Championship, 50-pound and under, and is currently attempting to defend his National Championship for the 1980 season in the 55-pound class, 10 years old and under.)

As we drove back to our home in Edmonds, Washington we reminisced about the rich experiences our family shared over the last few years and how Darren had developed into the strong, well coordinated wrestler he had become even at the age of eight.

"Boy! It sure is a good thing we know about rebound exercise, isn't it, Daddy," exclaimed Wendie.

"Yeah!" agreed Darren, "I'm glad the other wrestlers didn't know about it!"

"Well, you could sure tell the difference between his balance and his opponents'," remarked Wendie.

"I didn't really realize it made that much difference until we watched others his age," commented Bonnie.

"Dad," Darren said, "remember when we performed at the Marriott Hotel in Chicago?"

"And remember when we were in the Indy 500 parade," Wendie said, "and how you jumped up under the bridge and how you hung onto the beam?"

"Yes," I said, answering both of them at the same time.

They were recalling the tour sponsored by the Marriott Corporation when we traveled the United States putting on trampoline shows for Farrell's Ice Cream Parlour Restaurants. How could any of us forget those exciting nine months when our home was a 28-foot Executive Motor Home and their school teachers were their mom and dad.

By the time we returned home from that tour, Darren at five years of age and Wendie at nine, were real troupers. They had participated in more than 500 trampoline performances in high schools, Jr. highs and elementary schools. Most shows ended with standing ovations. Those were truly memorable and exciting performances. Up north, in Seattle and Portland, we performed in the gymnasiums or auditoriums of schools;

down south in Los Angeles and Houston out in the school yard or on football fields.

The 45-minute shows were practically the same each time, and we all had our responsibilities and parts. Darren demonstrated basic trampolining, and Wendie performed trampoline feats that high school students wished they could do. Wendie and I did a comedy trampoline routine that left audiences laughing hysterically. Each show ended with advance trampolining, which included the double somersaults, double twists, the suicide dive, and fliffises (double somersaults with twists).

Bonnie, the show's chief critic, managed the children backstage and handled all minute details and unexpected emergencies during performances. Our audiences saw us perform in basement gymnasiums in Pendleton, Oregon, on the roof of a five-story school in downtown San Francisco, on blacktop school yards and high school football fields in California. We dodged bad

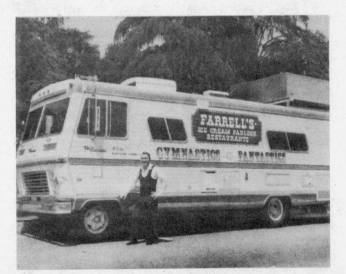

winter weather in Oklahoma and Arkansas; and our names were on marquees of shopping centers in Alabama. We suffered the heat and humidity of outdoor performances in New Orleans and Miami, and even survived New York's Staten Island traffic with our motorhome.

Our tour route took us through Ohio and Michigan. In Indiana we performed on national television, bouncing on a trampoline on an Indy 500 parade float traveling three miles an hour while we attempted to stay in the middle of the trampoline. We were well received in Denver where there are more trampolines per capita than any other place in the nation. Our tour climaxed in Salt Lake City, nine months after it started in Seattle; 500 shows and half a million people later. Neither Darren, Wendie, Bonnie nor I missed a single performance.

Returning to the great Northwest, we could now consider ourselves seasoned troupers, all. Darren had to learn how to write his name early on that tour so he could sign autographs after performances. The autograph would often be backwards, but it was his autograph. Before the tour, Wendie had been able to control three back somersaults in swing (back somersaults with only one bounce in between). By the end of the tour, she was doing twenty-four back somersaults in swing, and throwing full twisting back somersaults.

Our trip from Salt Lake City to Seattle, after our tour, was exhilarating. We basked in the sense of accomplishment of a job well done. We had seen the nation from Disneyland to Disneyworld, from Seattle to Florida, and now we were going back to buy a home, settle down, and live like other people live.

Now, after the national wrestling competitions, we were again heading back to our Seattle home. And once

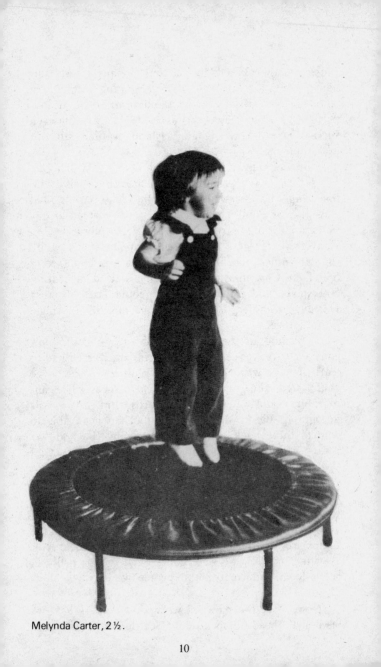

Melynda Carter, 2 ½.

again the same sense of accomplishment filled us. The air was electric, and we tingled with the success of Darren's accomplishments on the mat.

"Do you remember the day before Thanksgiving when we had to perform five shows and then drive to the airport in time to catch the airplane?" Darren reminisced.

"Yeah," answered Wendie, her own memory awakened, "and remember the time in Los Angeles when the wind was blowing so hard we had to jump into it just to stay in the middle of the trampoline?"

"Yeah! That was fun," said Darren.

"Mother, remember when we climbed Camel Back Mountain just outside Phoenix?" asked Wendie.

"I could never forget that," said Bonnie. "We were all tied together with that long rope and I was so afraid that one of us would fall and pull the others down."

"But you liked it on top, didn't you Mother?" asked Darren.

"Yes," said Bonnie, "especially when I found that the other side of the mountain was a gentle walk down."

"Will Melynda be sad that she doesn't have these memories?" Darren asked me.

"No," I said, "Melynda is only two. She has plenty of time for her own memories."

After our national tour, we had found a comfortable split level house on almost an acre of land; it had a little horse barn out back and a stream running through the middle of the pasture almost year round. After we moved in and the kids started school, Melynda came to bless our home. We were finally living the way other people lived. Wendie and Darren were attending school a quarter of a mile away, Bonnie had a new baby to love, dress and cherish, and I had my lawn to mow and weeds to pull. We were finally like a normal family — just like everybody else on the block — or were we?

I believe my first indication that my children were different was when Wendie was in sixth grade. She came home from school and nonchalantly informed us that she had just beaten all the sixth grade boys in arm wrestling.

"That's wonderful, Wendie," I complimented with mixed emotion wondering what the heck my daughter was doing arm wrestling the boys.

The next indication came when Darren wanted to go out for wrestling. I don't believe there is anything he could have wanted that would have made me happier. But it was very hard to believe that a second grade boy had the mental and physical capacity to learn the intricate and challenging art that had paid for my college education at Oklahoma State University and the University of Utah more than a dozen years earlier. A few quick pointers from Dad on the front room rug and Darren and I were off to talk to the coaches who, I thought, had to be a strange combination of babysitter and school yard fight instructor. I really wasn't surprised when the several coaches were impressed as Darren threw the "fireman's carry" on me in the middle of the mat exactly as I had instructed him. They immediately assumed that Darren had previous wrestling experience, and that, somehow at the age of seven, he was already an "old timer".

Before the first wrestling session ended, I found myself volunteering as one of the coaches to protect Darren's instant reputation. I must admit that we had a few more sessions on the front room rug where we went over some of the finer points I had learned during my wrestling career. I was pleasantly rewarded by Darren's ability to properly coordinate his muscles to execute even some of the finer wrestling moves. All that season,

Darren exhibited phenomenal balance, coordination, timing, speed, endurance, and strength for a seven year old. And although I was pleased as punch with his success, I pitied his seven and eight year old opponents simply because they were clearly no match for him.

To say that I was proud of the physical accomplishment of my children is an understatement. Darren won a first place gold medal in the Washington State Kids' Wrestling Championship for the 40-pound class of eight years and under, which was a mere formality. I apologetically told Darren that maybe next year there would be better competition. Wendie won the Washington State Jr. Olympic Trampoline Championship with no problem at all and went on to come in third behind two eighteen year old boys in the Regional Junior Olympics.

No one could know the thrilling experiences we shared when we, as a family, went into schools and performed trampoline exhibitions as the "Gymnastics Fantastics!"

Passing through Tacoma, northward on I-5 in our motorhome, I remember thinking to myself, "What a beautiful life we have working together as a family, helping one another with our accomplishments, and sharing dreams. How blessed we are! Why us?"

I was thirty-six years old and still able to do more than 100 one-arm push-ups. My mind flashed through the innersanctum of my private physician's office. I vividly recalled his surprised expression when he calculated my resting pulse rate at thirty-nine. I remember the exhilarating feeling leaving his office that day — thinking to myself that this is the age when most young executives begin to fall apart physically. It almost seemed unfair that I should be able to make money, have a meaningful relationship with my family, and remain physically fit without even trying! It was almost like make-believe.

"Daddy, when are we going to Disneyland again?" asked Darren, interrupting my thoughts.

"How about next year," I answered without hesitating. "We'll book school assemblies all the way from Seattle to Los Angeles and back, and just take off for two weeks the way we did it in '73. Only this time I'll be able to give lectures on rebound exercise in the evenings." That announcement met with cheers from everyone. Even Melynda clapped and cheered, although she didn't know what she was excited about.

"Rebound exercise," I thought to myself. "How time changes things! A year ago, the phrase didn't even exist!" It was really strange how we just took for granted the strength and coordination of each member of the family before I met Jerry. In fact, I don't remember ever in my life making a direct attempt to develop physical strength. Nor do I remember ever suggesting to my family that they consider strength an important attribute. I'm sure part of it was because we were never really concerned about developing strength; it always seemed to be there. Throughout my high school and college athletic career, although I won three state wrestling championships while other wrestlers were pumping iron trying to become strong, I never participated in a strength program. I preferred spending my time doing trampoline tricks. And because I never met any opponent on the wrestling mat that I considered as physically strong as myself, I discounted the need for a muscle development program. It's strange how we are blind to the obvious and how we take for granted blessings we don't have to work for.

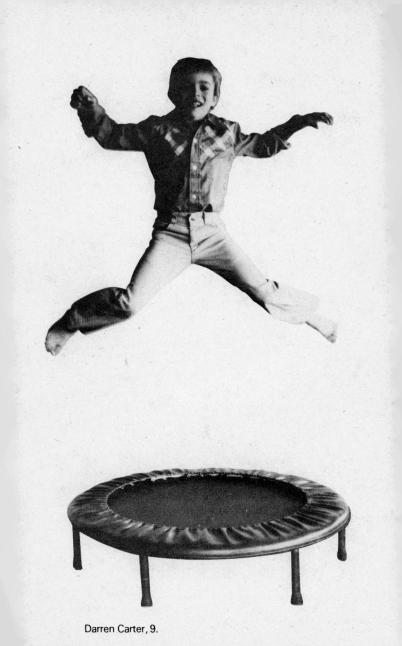

Darren Carter, 9.

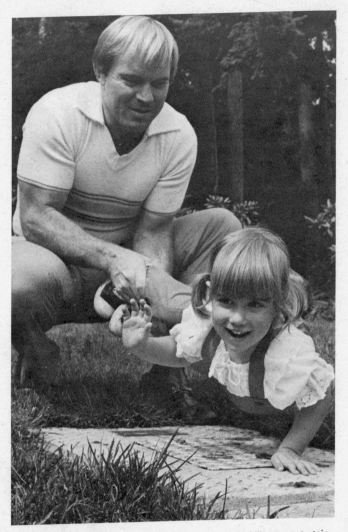

"And last but not least, Carter's daughter, Melynda, likes to entertain the neighborhood with one-armed pushups of her own. Melynda, mind you, is only three years old."

— *from Young Athlete, April 1980*

Chapter II
A Dream and a Dreamer

"Al."

"Yes, Bonnie."

"Telephone."

I still remember that call in early November, 1976.

"It's Bill Dearinger," explained Bonnie, "He wants to talk to you about a trampoline show for his church group, I think."

"That's strange," I thought. We had just performed for them about two months before.

"Hi, Bill. This is Al. May I help you?"

"Hi, Al. I would like to compliment you and your family on the great trampoline performance you gave us."

"Thanks," I said, wondering why he was thanking me two months later.

"Because you're so involved in trampolining, I'd like to come over and show you something I'm sure you and your family would really be interested in," he said.

Now, that sounded like a salesman's opener if I ever heard one.

"What is it?" I asked, wondering how to prevent him from wasting my time on something I wouldn't be interested in.

"Well," he said, "it's a piece of equipment used for exercise. I think you'll really enjoy it."

Now, that's really silly, I thought. Why would

anybody be trying to interest me in exercise equipment. That's the last thing I need. My whole vocation is exercise.

"Bill, there's nothing better than trampolining for keeping in shape," I replied defensively.

"That may be true," he said, "but you can't use it in your house. I've got a small, round exercise unit that you can bounce on right in your frontroom."

The thought of a small trampoline used in the frontroom hit me two different ways. I remembered when I used to sell Slim-Gyms; the only way to beat the convenience of the Slim-Gyms was to put a small trampoline in your recreation room or bedroom.   I remember thinking, "One of these days, somebody will perfect this concept and make a lot of money with it."

My second reaction was how in the world could anybody jump on a trampoline in a living room without either denting the ceiling with his skull or hitting the floor through the mat — or both!

I still wanted neither to buy anything nor to tangle with a salesman; but I had a responsibility to myself and to others who might ask my professional opinion of this exercise unit.

"Do you have that piece of equipment in your home now?" I asked.

"Yes, I do," answered Bill, "and my whole family uses it every day."

"Why don't I come over to your place and look at it?" I asked.

"Great!" he exclaimed. "When can you make it?"

"How about fifteen minutes?"

"We'll be waiting for you," he said.

I hung up, kissed Bonnie and told her I'd be back in an hour or so.

I remember that my mind raced a hundred miles an hour as I drove toward Bill's place. It would be fantastic if somebody had finally solved all the problems in marketing a safe in-home unit. The device would have to be strong enough for the heaviest family member, and yet resilient enough for children to use. It would have to be low enough to be safe for grandma and grandpa, yet high enough to not "bottom out", or hit the floor, as someone jumped up and down. It would also have to be small enough so children wouldn't mistake it for a trampoline to do tricks on, yet large enough so that even a clumsy person would not fall.

I had already decided, several years ago, that if a unit were to be used for exercise, it could not be used for tricks. That meant the mat surface had to be parallel to the floor and not otherwise adjustable. Mini-trampolines have an adjustable mat so the trajectory or direction of the bounce can be altered according to the mat angle. But above all, the unit would have to be of highest quality, and I would accept no compromise on that point.

I'd been performing on the very best equipment — the Nissen Goliath trampoline — for more than twenty years, and I was very choosy about the quality of equipment to which I trusted my life and health.

By the time I had arrived at Bill's house, I'd already determined that no piece of equipment could possibly meet all my requirements. I'd tear Bill's contraption apart and explain why it was dangerous, shoddy, frail, or nothing more than a toy.

I could see the thing from Bill's doorway as he opened the door. It stood less than a foot off the ground on six round chrome legs and looked as if it were trying to hide by blending in with the other furniture.

Bill and I exchanged brief greetings — my critical eyes glued to the equipment. I went over, picked it up, turned it over and attacked its soft underbelly fully expecting to find a fatal flaw. Surprisingly, I was impressed with the solid, quality construction. I carefully studied the stitching, it was strong. And I had to admit that the springs were of better quality than those on my $2,000.00 professional trampoline. I turned the unit over, set it on its sturdy chrome legs, stood back and looked at its profile.

Ah-ha! I thought, "There's the flaw! It's too low. No adult could bounce on that without hitting the floor. In fact, the fabric would probably rip out with any amount of use at all.

I asked Bill if he had ever bottomed out on this unit.

"No," he replied without hesitation. Then he just doesn't know how to bounce, I thought. A few of my quick, solid bounces will show Bill how dangerous this thing could be to a person's spinal column when I hit the floor.

I took off my shoes and stepped in the middle of the machine. It was surprisingly resilient. After a couple of quick, easy bounces, I put my heels together and thrust them into the mat. My attack was met by an equal and opposite force that catapulted me into the air. I hadn't hit the floor!

"That's impressive," I said, employing candor to save face.

"Are those legs adjustable?" I asked, picking the unit up and answering the question myself. Each leg was solidly welded to the round steel frame.

"It's a good thing those legs won't come off," I said, trying to sound as professional as possible.

"Why?" he asked.

"Can you imagine trying to jump on one of these things if one of the legs wasn't properly attached?" I said.

I felt a curious, rising anticipation. It was as if somebody had read my mind and developed this machine according to my specifications. Could this possibly be the first individualized rebound machine to meet my rigid requirements? I inspected it again and observed how the springs were uniquely triangulated.

Of course! I thought, no wonder I can't bottom out. Each spring protects the other by not allowing its neighboring spring to extend to its maximum length. What a fantastic idea! I wished I had thought of that. The person who put this thing together really knew what he was doing.

"Who's manufacturing these units, Bill?" I asked.

"One of the executives is here in town," he answered.

"When can I see him?" I tried to camouflage my excitement.

"Well, we've got a public meeting next Thursday, and . . . "

"I'd like to see him before next Thursday," I said, cutting him off, " . . . privately."

"Well, he's very busy," Bill began.

"Bill, if you want me to get involved in any way, you'll get me an appointment to see him immediately!" My facade was gone.

I left the Dearinger home excited by the possibilities of this amazing machine!

Two days later, Jerry Hinkle walked into my office at noon, as previously arranged. He was tall, had black wavy hair and a perpetual smile that radiated a glowing personality. His trim 210 pound frame said "former athlete!" Dressed in a tasteful, light blue suit and spit-polished shoes, he gave the impression of a Dale Carnegie Course honor graduate.

"I'm Jerry Hinkle," he said in the thick accent of an Arkansas farmer turned professional salesman about thirty years ago.

"Just because we talk funny don't mean we think slow," he's quipped many times since that initial introduction. Our planned half-hour luncheon at Jimbo's turned into a two and one-half hour soul-search involving an exciting concept we held in common but approached from entirely different directions.

He told me about the experiences his friends were having with this new, fun and easy way to exercise. I confirmed his claims by relating the experiences my family and I had shared in our years as trampolinists. He graphically unveiled a panorama of the potential of this revolutionary new exercise concept — his exercise machine playing the major role. Then, he substantiated his dream with amazing but believable stories of aging ladies looking younger and invalids walking again.

He talked about the necessity of quality workmanship and materials, and expressed a genuine desire for consumer value for dollars spent. He personified the old-fashioned idea of integrity in a man's word being his bond and his handshake as good as his contract.

As I sat across the table listening to him unfold his hopes for the future, I knew I was listening to a man deeply concerned about the health and well-being of his fellowmen. If honesty, loyalty, and integrity receive their fair value, surely this man would one day receive royal compensation.

Jerry knew that this type of exercise was fun, easy, refreshing, and often the only exercise the elderly could enjoy; but he was not a trampolinist. I was certain he was unaware of the fullest potential of this type of exercise, and I told him so.

"Jerry, do you know what you've got here?" I asked.

"Yes," he said, "a gold mine. It's a fun, easy way to exercise in the convenience of your own home."

"Even if that were all it is, Jerry, it's a great idea; but it's more than that. You have just made it possible for almost every living person to take advantage of the most efficient, effective form of exercise yet devised by man!" I said.

I suddenly realized I was quoting a statement I had memorized when I was fourteen years old. Bill Stallings, my gymnastic coach, made that statement to all the first year gymnasts in a lecture before our first written gymnastic test. The lecture and test were given to us in the interest of safety. I remember studying hard for that particular test because we weren't allowed on any of the school's gymnastic equipment until after we had passed it. I remember, as coach Stallings made that statement, how I questioned that trampolining could be a better exercise than other gymnastic events.

"What do you mean?" asked Jerry.

"Are you aware that it strengthens every muscle in your body?" I asked.

"Well, I hadn't heard that," he answered, "how can jumping up and down do anything for the arms?"

"Well, it does," I blurted out. "I've never lifted weights in my life, and look at me. I've got a very strong healthy body, and at thirty-six I can still do over 100 one-arm push-ups."

"Do you mean that?" Jerry questioned.

"Of course! And that's just the beginning," I answered.

"Is there some way you can document those statements? If you can, we'll have the hottest piece of exercise equipment on the market!" he exclaimed. "Will you personally endorse this method of exercise?"

"Certainly!" I said. "But you need more than an endorsement. You need exhaustive research and full documentation so you can tell the whole world what rebounding is all about."

"Can you get that information for me?" he asked.

"I don't see why not," I said, "it's probably already available in libraries if you know where to look."

"Well, we would make good use of any reference material you could locate to back up your theories," he said.

We left Jimbo's that day both tingling with enthusiasm — Jerry with anticipation of greater insight to his exercise unit, and I with the desire to prove to the world something I'd come to know through more than twenty years of experience on trampolines.

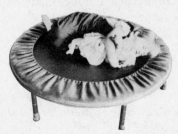

Chapter III
Discovery of a Void

The next day, I was in the library checking out books on health, physiology, human anatomy, aerobics and various exercises. Among them were books on trampolining, jogging, jumping rope, and texts on physical education. My concern, that day, was merely finding from which text books I wanted to quote. I fully expected to find all the information about what happens to the physical body while on the trampoline. After all, hadn't I received this information from my trusted gymnastic instructors? And where had they received their information?

That evening, after the children were in bed, I began to study the stack of books on top of the desk in front of me. Among them was one loaned to me by Jerry; *Physiology of Exercise,* by Morehouse, PhD., and Miller, M.D. I was immediately impressed with their approach to the subject of exercise and its effect on the health of the human body. On pages 220 and 221, I found exercises listed according to the number of calories burned per hour. The list started with "sleeping" and ended with, "horizontal running at 18.9 miles per hour."

Imagine my disappointment when, after going over the list three or four times, I couldn't find trampolining among the exercises. Surely, I thought, this must be an oversight by the authors, because everyone knows of the effect trampolines have had on our youth in elementary, junior high, and high schools. At one time we had NCAA competition; and even today we have national and world trampoline competition.

I concluded that what I needed was a physiology book with a larger list of exercises. One of the books I checked out was the *International Guide to Fitness and Health*, by Larson & Michelman. On the front cover it boasted that it was, "from the latest research of the International Committee on Standardization, which included the fields of medicine, nutrition and physical education. Here are the most authoritative techniques for planning a really workable, enjoyable, individual exercise program." Surely this book would have what I was looking for. I found their list beginning on page 50 and continuing for the next five pages. Their exercises were listed alphabetically beginning with "archery" and ending with "yard work." This list of 133 physical "exercises" included such activities as "kite flying, putting practice, Jai alai, resting, tumbling, and even piloting a plane." But something was missing. Under the T's, I found no mention of trampolining!

Now, I wasn't just disappointed — I was hurt. If I were a baseball player, I could find my sport, but I was a trampolinist and mine wasn't there.

For the next two weeks, I searched every library I could find for any physiology book that even mentioned trampolining. None! I also pulled out all the books I could find on trampolining written by trampolinists, but, to my amazement, even these books made no mention of what actually happens to the body while jumping up and down. Even the Encyclopedia Brittanica and Americana failed.

Page 294, Volume 19, 1978 Edition of World Book Encyclopedia

Trampoline. "It is an elastic canvas or net bed used in gymnastics, especially tumbling. It is often

26

called a bouncing or bounding table. It is usually about eight feet or two meters wide and fifteen feet or five meters long. Springs or cord anchor the bed to a metal frame of table height."

Volume 26, Page 926, Encyclopedia Americana, Copyright 1977

Trampoline. "An elevated resilient constructed bed or mat used by gymnasts, acrobats and others as a performing surface. A spring or rubber suspension system anchor the beds to a table type steel frame, the sides of which are padded to protect the user from injury. The springs attach to the bed and cause the performer to continue to bound upward. The activity that takes place on the apparatus is called trampolining or rebound tumbling . . . .

To my knowledge, there has been no study whatever about what happens to the body when one is bouncing on the trampoline. The trampoline has been a platform for gymnastic tricks — and that's all.

In desperation, I finally called The Nissen Corporation in Cedar Rapids, Iowa. Surely they could lead me to the proper book, if one existed. After all, according to the *Guinness Book of Records,* it was George Nissen who invented the trampoline in 1936, and it was Nissen equipment I had been working on for the past twenty years. I even had use of the Nissen Watts line, should I need any information. My call went straight through to the top, and I talked at some length to Robert J. Bevenour, Executive Vice President of The Nissen Corporation. To my dismay, I learned he faced the same problem. He did say that he would send me everything in his file on the subject; he requested that, should I find further information, I reciprocate by sending it to directly to him.

Well, I thought, The Nissen Corporation has been the

leader in the trampoline industry and is the world's largest gymnastic equipment manufacturing company today. If it doesn't have any information on the benefits of trampolining, then I must have been fooling myself for all these years.

Discouraged, I decided it was best to tell Jerry that no such health benefit existed. At least he could sell his exercise equipment as a good alternative to jogging.

Jerry and his wife, Maple, listened to me as I explained my disappointment.

"Well, just write up a short page of how you feel," suggested Maple. "At least that's more than we have now."

I felt I'd really let them down; but I agreed to write up something, and left completely dejected and unfulfilled. I thought, "How could I be so self-centered to think that my particular form of exercise was better than any other?"

I was practically sleepless the next week. As I began to return books to the library. I thumbed through the pages searching for answers that weren't there; then I began to ask myself,

"If rebounding isn't the best exercise, then what is? If there is a best exercise, why is it better than the others?"

I still had the last book I was returning. The library would close in an hour. Before turning it in, I sat down and began to study the list of exercises in the *International Guide to Fitness and Health* one last time. I studied the categories to find out which one was best; and I remembered turning to page 49 and reading this:

"Before beginning any program, you have your doctor check your general health. If there are any physical disabilities, these should be added to the other factors previously discussed in determining your program and activities. Once you have

determined the desirable channel for your purposes, then read Chapter 6 and select your program and activities. There is a wide range of activities from which to select within each channel.

Now consider your objective: (a) physical fitness and work capacity, (b) general health, (c) physical appearance, (d) physical recreation. Select your objective after carefully reviewing all the objectives, their subdivisions, and the programs designed for them. (See Tables XVI, XVII, XVIII, XIX. Refer also to the Tables in Chapter 4.)

"The channels include the following cardiac risk conditions: (a) normal, (b) some risk, and (c) high risk. Refer to Table II and your medical examination to determine your proper program.

"Determine your body weight: (a) normal weight, (b) overweight or underweight, (c) obese weight levels. Refer to Table II, Chapter 4 for proper placement.

"Determine your tension level: (a) normal, (b) tense. Refer to Table II, Chapter 4.

"After you find your proper exercise channel, use Tables XVI, XVII, XVIII, or XIX to provide guides for your exercise program. Consider:
1. Dietary needs.
2. Exercise requirements for the channel. These guides will indicate the function, system, and organs of the body of particular importance in achieving the goal.
3. The emphasis required to achieve your goal (e.g., General Endurance: 1, 2, or 3).
4. Any special needs — dietary and/or corrective-adaptive exercises.

"Now read Chapter 6 for suggestions about the specific activities."

We are dangerously over-eager to have experts tell us exactly what to do and exactly what the outcome will be if we follow their instructions explicitly. To many, exercise has become a science. Amazed, I laid the book down.

"What has this country come to?" I asked myself. According to what I'd just read, a person would have to be an accountant, a scientist, or a robot just to get a good exercise program. And if that's the case, how in the world did we survive until we knew how to read! What about strong, healthy savages in parts of this world where they live and die without even hearing the word "exercise"?

I began thinking that maybe I had missed the boat! I didn't realize exercise was so complicated. Surely there was a better answer!

I pulled out a piece of paper and began to write down everything all these exercises have in common. Half way through the list, I stopped. I felt as if someone had just turned on a light inside my brain. I flipped the next two pages and scanned the exercises.

"That's it!"

I jumped up and started pacing around the table, my mind moving a million miles an hour recalling everything I had read in the last couple of weeks.

"It's so simple! Why hasn't anybody thought of it before? If someone has, why hasn't he said so? All exercises have one thing in common: every exercise in some way is related to the earth's gravitational pull! No, not, related — opposes the gravitational pull of the earth. That's it! **The common denominator of all exercises is opposition to the gravitational pull of the earth!**

I went over the exercises quickly, one by one, to see if this checked. What about push-ups? Yes, we are pushing away from gravity. Chin-ups? Of course! We are pulling our bodies away from the gravitational pull of the earth. And sit-ups? That's gravity pulling down on the torso as we move away from it. What about leg-lifts? We are opposing gravity with the other end of our bodies. And weight lifting? Here, it was easy to see that what man had done was to devise a method by which he could oppose gravity by controlling the mass that he pulled or lifted away from gravity. In fact, weight, by definition is: mass X gravity.

Even the aerobic exercises, such as walking, jogging or running, depend on the gravitational pull of the earth to be effective.

To walk, the first thing one does is move his center of gravity off the base until he starts falling forward; then he has to take a step to keep from being completely pulled down by the gravitational force.

Even swimming is directly influenced by the gravitational pull of the earth. Although the body appears to be defying the law of gravity through buoyancy while swimming, it is the gravitational pull of the earth that makes water dense enough to establish resistance to the muscular movements of the swimmer. Every exercise listed causes the body to oppose gravity in some way — even trampolining — and it wasn't listed among the exercises. But, to me, trampolining seemed to do a better job.

"Mr. Carter, we're closing now."

How dare that librarian break into my private discovery!

"Okay. I'll need to check this book out again, and this one, and this one."

I was starting my research all over again; only this time I was getting somewhere.

My next stop: Jerry and Maple Hinkle's home. Somehow, I was going to prove that rebounding was not just fun and easy, but that it was also extremely effective.

The next few weeks, Bonnie and I spent every spare moment, and even some we couldn't spare, writing and rewriting the manuscript of *Rebound to Better Health*. The book began to take shape; arguments were labored, but, we felt, convincing. We knew there had to be something more to it than just opposition to gravity, because all exercises shared that common, everpresent force.

Finally, after several nights of writing and rewriting, I felt again that I was spinning my wheels accomplishing nothing. I was still grasping for something that wasn't there. I began to have thoughts like:

Maybe this is why no one has written about what happens to the physical body while jumping up and down.

One night, after midnight, I was alone at my desk. I felt trapped by my commitment and not able to do anything about it. I went over to the set of encyclopedias, the *New Book of Knowledge*, and looked up "gravity" to see if I could find anything else that would bolster our position. I found "gravity" on page 320 in volume 7. Gloom descended as I read:

"For 300 years scientists have studied gravitation. They can measure its strength and tell other things about it. But the question, 'What is gravitation,' is still a mystery."

I continued reading the next paragraph,

"In 1911, the famous scientist, Albert Einstein, developed the new idea of gravitation. He showed that gravitation and acceleration produced the same effects. There is no way to tell gravitation from acceleration."

I looked up from the book in a half daze,

"That's it!" I said to myself. "That's what was missing! Bonnie, I've found it!"

I leaped from my chair, grabbed the book and ran upstairs to our bedroom where Bonnie lay sleeping.

"I found the key! I found what we've been looking for! And it was in our basement all the time!"

"You found what?" asked Bonnie, not quite awake.

"Listen! There's more than one force we are working with!" I exclaimed.

"Let's talk about it in the morning," she said as she rolled over and pulled the covers up over her head.

"No! I've got to talk to you now!" I exclaimed. "How can you sleep when I'm so excited?"

"I can't, so I'll listen," she said, sitting up. "Now, what did you find in our basement?"

"The answer! We've been talking about opposing gravity. Acceleration is a completely different force, but the body can't tell the difference between acceleration and gravity. Therefore, if you accelerate vertically, like in a rocket ship or on a trampoline, you develop a greater G force. And because the body can't tell the difference, it accepts acceleration as gravity!"

For the next two hours, we brainstormed, and things began to unscramble and fall into place.

The next day, I borrowed *Medical Physiology*, by Guyton, from Dr. Darryl Rogers, D.D.S. Bonnie's brother; a section entitled, "Space Physiology," verified what we had just discovered. It points out that the federal government has spent millions of dollars of our money studying the effects of acceleration and deceleration on the human body, both horizontally and vertically. Now we had **three** forces that we could identify — gravity, acceleration, and deceleration

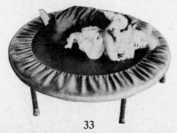

Chapter IV
Three Powerful Horses

Flying across the United States recently, at 37,000 feet, in a very comfortable climate controlled, pressurized DC-10, I became acutely aware of an interesting fact. I couldn't see the earth in the darkness of night, and, for the moment, the only thing that existed was the pod in which a few fellow humans were casually eating, snoozing, reading, and chatting with one another. But our every move was influenced by the same physical forces we contend with while we are standing on the earth.

The theory of universal gravitation presented to us by Sir Isaac Newton explains that the same force holding the moon and planet in orbit is also present in the aircraft holding the liquid in my glass in place. That theory states that every body is subjected to gravity. The liquid in my glass pulls as hard on the earth as the earth pulls on the liquid. For example, the moon's gravity pulls on the earth as the earth's gravity pulls on the moon. This is evidenced by the moon's ability to influence the high tides as it orbits around the earth. There is a greater gravitational pull on water directly below the moon, which causes a swelling or an accumulation of large amounts of water, creating a high tide.

Sir Isaac Newton's theory of universal gravitation encompasses the inner-relationship and movement of every particle of the universe. However, we live on the earth, and our bodies are primarily affected by the earth's gravitational pull. Newton found that the strength of gravitation depends on several things: **First,** it depends on how much matter a body contains. A body with much matter receives much gravitation. For example, the earth has more matter than the moon, so the earth's gravitational pull is stronger than the moon's. **Second,** the strength of gravitation depends on the distance between the bodies. It is stronger between bodies close together. Newton worked out this equation for gravitation; it gives the strength of gravitation between two bodies:

$$f = \frac{m_1 \times m_2}{r^2}$$

In the equation, f stands for the force of gravitation. The amount of matter in one body is m_1; the amount of matter in the other body is m_2. r_2 is the distance between the bodies.

DISTANCE = 1 — FORCE OF GRAVITY $= \frac{M_1 \times M_2}{r \times r} = \frac{1}{1 \times 1} = 1$

DISTANCE = 2 — FORCE OF GRAVITY $= \frac{1}{2 \times 2} = \frac{1}{4}$

DISTANCE = 3 — FORCE OF GRAVITY $= \frac{1}{3 \times 3} = \frac{1}{9}$

According to Newton's theory, if the mass of the two bodies remains the same as the distance doubles, the gravitational pull will be reduced by one fourth. If the distance between triples, the gravitational pull will be reduced by one-ninth.

On the earth, two other things determine the strength of the gravitational pull: (a) distance from the center of the earth; and (b) spin of the earth. Therefore, a very slight difference exists in the gravitational pull at various places on the earth. For our purposes, although this difference is measurable, it is not important. '

Gravity is pulling on all particles of the atmosphere; therefore, all of us are subjected to the atmospheric pressure. We live at the bottom of a massive ocean of air, or atmosphere that has been captured by the gravitational pull of the earth. The air, or atmosphere, is pulled down toward the center of the earth and applies pressure to everything in it at 14.7 pounds per square inch of exposed surface at sea level. The atmospheric pressure on the earth dictates the amount of pressure inside our bodies. It influences every cell throughout the entire body. Pressure inside each cell must be between 6 mm Hg and 1 mm Hg of the outside pressure of each cell. Otherwise, the cell wall would collapse or rupture. ² The body has the amazing ability to adjust to the various amounts of pressure we experience here on the earth. But any time man ventures too far from the earth's surface, whether down in the ocean or to the moon, he must take his environment, or atmospheric pressure, with him. Although the cabin in the airplane was pressurized, I still had to swallow several times during our descent to equalize the pressure on the inside of my body to that on the outside.

Therefore, gravity directly influences every cell in the body in two ways: (a) atmosphere pressure pushing in from all directions, and (b) direct gravitational pull on every cell. **Gravity is the most important and constant physical force of our existence.** Gravity is our teacher, our coach, our doctor, and our chief opposition. Gravity develops a weak baby into a strong child. It helps the lame to walk and the blind to see. It actually has the capability of making the old feel younger again. As we learn more about it, gravity teaches us to fly to the moon and back. It is universal and constant — an eternal law. Gravity is one of those laws that were decreed in heaven before the foundation of the earth, and when we understand and use this law properly, blessings of health, wisdom, and great knowledge are ours for the asking. [3]

Gravity is a very impressive force; but there is another law just as important and everlasting as gravity. In fact, it is impossible to use gravity without it. The only way the law of gravitation can be used to develop strength is by opposing it in some way. The earth would not remain in its orbit around the sun without centrifugal force opposing gravity. Man would never fly to the moon without spending great amounts of energy opposing gravity. No rivers could exist without some force moving the moisture from the ocean to the tops of the mountains. Samson would never have been strong if he hadn't first lifted his head from his infant crib to look around, thereby beginning the process of strengthening his body. Thus, we have the answer to the secret of the construction of the pyramids. We have identified a law that is just as important as gravity itself. It is the universal law of strength to have an opposition in all things. To gain strength, health, wisdom, or knowledge, man must have an opposition. To use the law of gravity, for strength, man must oppose it. **You have to have an opposition to develop strength. Where there is no opposition, there is no strength!**

Born into this environment, we therefore have one or two choices: either oppose the gravitational pull or give in to it. Earth's constant gravitational pull attempts to claim its own. It is always there to welcome man to give up and fold into a compact mass; to surrender to the constant urge, to assume constrictive movements, symbolizes fatigue, withdrawal, defeat, and resignation. The catatonic patient who resumes the fetal position is an example of its most extreme form. The expansive, outward, upward movements of a ballet dancer, a gymnast, a trampolinist, or an athlete who seeks to obtain freedom of movement through exercise symbolizes man's aspirations to advance, to rise farther above the earth, to challenge, to live, to achieve, to oppose the downward pull of gravity. [4]

A newborn's first challenge is to lift his head away from the force that constantly pulls him down. Gravity, then, by opposition, teaches that child to crawl, walk, run, jump, play, and throw balls. Against that constant opposition, that child stands up and becomes an adult.

A child starts life with a basic capability for movement and a set of movement characteristics distinguishable, to some degree, soon after birth. Patterns of movement, which are developed in the human infant during the first three years, are organized specifically with reference to gravitational forces acting on the body in relation to the spaces, objects, and surfaces in his environment.

Man's upright posture governs the way he experiences the world. The vertical and horizontal axes of perceived space are established only with reference to gravity. His visual clues assist the postural ones. Because the very framework of perceived space is dependent on the need to maintain upright and correct equilibrium against the pull of gravity, the way man sees his world depends on his upright posture. For man to function properly, he must get right with the gravitational pull. [5]

Man's amazing body is designed to achieve equilibrium automatically after basic procedure is learned. Small sensory hairs in the inner ear are affected by the relationship between gravity and the position and movement of the head. The semi-circular ducts in the inner ear are the sense organs of dynamic equilibrium. They are responsible for initiating body-righting reflexes, or, in other words, making sure that the body is at right angles to the horizontal plane of the earth.

To coordinate the body position, there are superficial and deep nerve receptors in the feet and the rest of the body that relay to the control center the relationship of the body to the gravitational forces. Impulses from these widely located sensory receptors integrate and converge on a final pathway to bring about effective and coordinated responses of anti-gravity muscles. Strengthening these muscles by proper vigorous exercise enables us to retain or recover normal orientation in space. Equilibrium occurs when we can identify where we are relative to the gravitational pull of the earth. [6]

Now that we understand a little more about the effects of gravity, let's take a closer look at the two controlable forces, acceleration and deceleration.

When we want to go some place we get into our automobile, turn on the key, step on the accelerator, and move forward. We feel the force of acceleration pushing us back into the seat.

We step on the brake and we feel the force of deceleration pushing us forward.

A gun kicks because of the bullet's acceleration.

A carpenter drives a nail when the force of deceleration transfers from the head of a hammer to the nail.

Even though these three forces are separate and distinct, Einstein indicates that our bodies cannot tell the difference between acceleration, deceleration and gravity.

In a space physiology study, N.A.S.A. spent millions investigating the effects of these three forces on man.

Test pilots were strapped into jet sleds that ran on rails. The sleds were allowed to accelerate so fast that the men were subjected to an acceleration force nine and ten times that of gravity. This study was necessary to know that astronauts were able to withstand the seven G force during lift-off at Cape Kennedy. That meant that a 175 pound astronaut immediately after blast off would weigh 1225 pounds! (A "G" force is a measure of the amount of gravitational pull on an object at sea level.)

When the astronauts returned to earth, they experienced another increase in body weight. It happened when they opened their drag parachutes to slow their landing module down during re-entry into the earth's atmosphere. Their bodies increased in weight by at least 4½ G's. One of the G forces was gravity, but the other 3½ G's were deceleration. However, their bodies accepted them as an increase in gravity. '

I felt the force of acceleration when my DC-10 began to increase in velocity down the runway for takeoff. Although I was trying to lean forward to look out the window, the acceleration pushed me back into the seat. The force disappeared when we reached the cruising speed predetermined by our flight plan.

When the DC-10 touched down, my body strained against my seat belt until we had slowed sufficiently to turn and taxi.

Although we have studied the effects of these forces on our bodies, we haven't used this information to exercise.

As an example, when one does push-ups, he is exercising a portion of his body by:

1. opposing gravity with the extender muscles of his arms only;
2. accelerating the top of his body at the beginning of the push; and

3. decelerating only the top of his body at the bottom as his chest touches the floor.

But, have we ever heard a coach yell, "All right, let's oppose gravity a few more times"? No.

Or, "Come on guys. Accelerate." No.

Have you ever heard, "Get in there and decelerate"? Never.

I was explaining this concept to an audience in Pennsylvania when an Amish gentleman stood up and said, "Mr. Carter, what you are trying to tell us is that we have three natural forces available to us at no cost that we could use to exercise and keep healthy, but we haven't been harnessing them up right."

"What do you mean?" I inquired.

"Well, it is as if I had three powerful horses and I hooked them all up to the same plow with one pulling to the right and one pulling to the left and one straining straight ahead. I would have a hard time getting my plowing done, wouldn't I?"

"You have the idea exactly," I said. We have accepted the forces of acceleration and deceleration as parts of our environment. We have even learned to control them. But we haven't accepted the fact that we can drastically change the cellular environment of our bodies just by lining up these three forces all in one direction. Obviously, our Amish farmer will get more plowing done by making sure all three of his horses pull the same direction. Likewise, by lining up acceleration, deceleration and gravity, we will be able to use these forces more efficiently.

Now we cannot control gravity. We are only subjected to it, but we can control the other two forces. Let us line up acceleration and deceleration with gravity. That is the purpose of the rebounder.

As we stand still on a rebounder, every cell in the body is opposing gravity. This can be measured with a

"G" meter. Of course, we all know that a bathroom scale is a "G" meter. If you were to take the bathroom scale and put it on top of the rebounder under your feet, it would register 1G force as long as you stand still. However, something fascinating happens when you start to move up and down. At the bottom of the bounce, you no longer weigh one G, you weigh more! At the bottom of the bounce, the needle on the scale would register a greater G force because it would be registering the combined forces of gravity plus deceleration when your body stops its downward thrust and acceleration when the expanded springs of the rebounder contract and forces your body back up.

Acceleration + Deceleration + Gravity = Greater G Force!

Even without allowing your feet to leave the rebounder mat, the G force would increase to approximately 125%!

Try it! You will see what I mean.

It is vitally important to realize that every cell in your body is directly affected by that 25% increase in G force. Every cell is individually stressed by an increase of 25%.

If you ask a coach, doctor, or physical therapist, "What is the formula for cellular strength?" the answer would be, "controlled stress below the rupture threshold times repetition."

Bouncing on a rebounder stresses every cell over and over again approximately 100 times a minute. The reason for the repetition is that every cell in your body has the unique ability to automatically adjust to its environment. Stressing a cell just once will not cause that cell to adjust to a new environment. By stressing every cell over and over again, every cell will begin to adjust to a greater G force and thereby become stronger.

Question: Why oppose gravity with only part of your body by doing push-ups, pull-ups, or leg-lifts, if you are

43

able to oppose gravity, add acceleration and deceleration to every part of your body, all at once, simply by rebounding?

Thus we have the amazing theory of rebound exercise; and you can now begin to understand why it is the most efficient, effective form of exercise yet devised by man.

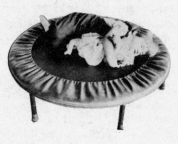

Chapter V
Rebound Exercise —
Past and Present

Today, more than ever before, the civilized world is in an exercise revolution. *Newsweek* recently published an article entitled, "Ready, Set, Sweat," in which the author reported on the jogging craze spreading all across the United States. *Better Homes and Gardens* recently had an eight-page tearout section on family fitness. Most major newspapers are carrying articles in which they admonish more stringent exercise habits. Jogging shoes and sweat clothes never sold faster; and "aerobics" is as common in social gatherings of stockbrokers, doctors, dentists, and executives as it is among the athletes. Sales of health spa memberships are at an all-time high, along with sales of bicycles and ski equipment. It is socially acceptable to talk about sweating, shin splints, Achilles tendon, aching backs, blisters, strains, sprains, and torn ligaments. The most popular person at a party is the one who can convincingly explain to his listeners why he is no longer jogging at 5:00 a.m. as he used to with the others.

Dr. Ken Cooper popularized the term "aerobics" in his books on exercise. He provides a point system for each type of accepted aerobic exercise so that an accountant or banker can now calculate the approximate amount of oxygen reaching his cells.

There seems to be as much controversy over exercise

now as the energy crisis question. It appears that the only way to solve the problem is to go back to the basics of exercise.

What is a good exercise? The human body is an intricate universe of organs, systems, muscles, bones, cells, enzymes and chemicals. Each is responsible for doing its own part for the good of the whole body. To function properly each has to do its own thing without endangering or harming any other part of the body. A good exercise would have to be a motion or activity that enhances the proper environment for healthy cells without infringing or endangering the existence or health of other healthy cells within the same body.

If we accept this definition, many sports and exercises do not qualify as good exercise. Football, basketball, soccer and all other contact sports where high possibility of injury to healthy cells exists, would have to be carefully analyzed. Although jogging has proven to be an excellent exercise for the cardiovascular system, it is, according to the experts, devastating to the skeletal structure.

Dr. George Sheehan, M.D., cardiologist and well known long distance runner and author of *Running and Being* states that jogging can be detrimental to the human body. In the *Executive Fitness Newsletter*, November 1977, Dr. Sheehan says the problem is not a medical one, but a structural one — almost architectural.

Sheehan points out that if your second toe is longer than your first toe, you may have what is called Morton's Foot, which is probably the most disabling of the common defects in the architecture of the foot, and causes it to break down in over-use. He cites Dudley Morton, the author of a book in 1935 titled, *The Human Foot*, and indicates that the function of the foot depends on two factors: a) structural stability supplied by the 26 bones and 112 ligaments that bind the bones together, and b) postural stability maintained by the short and the long muscles of the foot and leg. Any abnormality in the bone architecture or laxity of the ligaments can end in weak and inefficient feet. Imbalance, caused by the short heel cord or strong inflexible calf and thigh muscles, may put additional stress on the foot and arch. The foot adapts by either (a) bearing the most of the weight on the head of the second metatarsal causing a stress fracture, or (b) pronating the foot over the side and opening up a Pandora's Box of overuse injuries.

A year ago, when I mentioned the term "rebound exercise" to people, very few, if any, understood what I was talking about; but when I mentioned "trampolining," almost everyone had some understanding of the subject, and many were able to relate personal experience of their involvement with trampolining. Their stories began with how one learned to do a somersault in a physical education class or how one fell into the springs attempting a somersault. They ended with the time one could pay twenty-five cents for a half-hour at a trampoline center. There, all trampolines were in the ground, out in the open, and had little or no supervision.

Ever since the trampoline was commercially manufactured, in 1936 by George Nissen, rebound exercise has been available to the American public in some form or other. However, for the most part, the only people who took advantage of this marvelous exercise were gymnastic students. In fact, trampoline has never been really seriously considered as a form of exercise.

Trampolining was introduced in the armed services just before World War II. The Army, Navy, Air Force, Paratroopers, and Marines used the trampoline to develop balance, dexterity, coordination, rhythm, and timing; but it was most important in developing strong, tough, well developed physiques.

One of the major problems of trampolining, however, was that the exercise was so effective the participants were able to propel their bodies great distances with few muscles. It literally catapulted them into an environment to which they were not accustomed. Because it was so much fun and so easy, any untrained person was tempted to rebound to dangerous heights and to attempt gymnastic moves without proper gymnastic instruction.

Trampoline instruction was practically non-existent between 1960 and 1961 when trampoline centers were available to anyone living in or near even the smallest town anywhere in U.S.A. Those who used the trampoline came off huffing and puffing, but they paid very little attention to the amount or quality of exercise received. After all, who in the world would think about exercise when the activity was so much fun and so easy!

The past few years, trampolining has been under fire by insurance companies because of injuries to participants without proper supervision. I think the key word here is "proper" supervision. For example, if you go swimming and you see a person sitting up in the high chair by the side of the swimming pool, you literally bet your life that that person is a certified, qualified life guard. You take scuba diving lessons from a certified scuba diving instructor, learn to ski from a certified ski instructor, and learn golf from a golf pro. But trampoline instruction is different. Any adult in our school systems, regardless of his physical education background, can be asked to supervise the trampoline when it is in use. And even our physical education instructors often complete their schooling with a major in physical education and have less than ten total hours of trampoline experience. As the physical education instructor or the coach, he may teach trampolining to as many as thirty-five students at once. Most physical education majors study gymnastics for a period of eight weeks; and in that eight weeks they must concern themselves with various girls' and boys' gymnastic events. Twelve separate events must be studied in fewer than eight weeks!

Neither the trampoline industry nor our education system has demanded that trampoline instructors be certified. We made this demand in our football, basketball, baseball, track and practically every other sport, but not trampolining. Thus, although trampolining is possibly the best all around body conditioner, it is being expelled from our schools because insurance costs have become prohibitive. Trampolining should be part of our education system, but not without certified trampoline instructors. As soon as the trampoline industry develops a method of qualifying and certifying instructors, trampolining will become part of our physical education programs in the schools; but not before.

In August, 1977, I published the book, *Rebound to Better Health*. As soon as it came off the press, I sent this fifty page booklet to people I considered experts in the trampoline industry and the fields of physiology, visual therapy, and chiropractic. On September 26, 1977, I received a very cordial letter from Mr. Robert Bevenour, executive vice president of the Nissen Corporation of Cedar Rapids, Iowa, a subsidiary of the Victor Comptometer Corporation. The Nissen Corporation is the world's largest gymnastic equipment company, and, at one time, it outsold all other such companies combined. Mr. Bevenour's letter says:

> "Many thanks, Al . . . for sending me your very interesting booklet.
>
> "It was one of the best medically oriented treatises I have ever read on the benefits of trampolining. With the sport of trampolining now under fire, as you suggest, perhaps we should be mailing something like this with every trampoline.
>
> "What is your position on having some of this

used in the new United States Gymnastics Safety Association Trampoline Certification Manual? . . . It's been a big chore just getting the manual together, and it is deficient in the area of trampoline benefits. Could they use some of your contents?"

I was understandably thrilled to receive that letter. But more meaningful to me was the realization that if that small booklet was the best medically oriented treatise on rebound exercise that Bob Bevenour had ever read, how little information was indeed available about rebound exercise. In fact, to my knowledge, when I published *Rebound to Better Health,* that was the first time the term "rebound exercise" was ever in print!

That rebound exercise has been completely ignored does not alter the fact that it is the most convenient, effective, efficient, economical, fun, and easy form of exercise yet devised by man. This has been brought about by the development of the small, springy fabric platform known as the rebounder. Now, for the first time, rebound exercise is available to any household. Entire families are taking turns getting in shape, toning and tightening their muscles, increasing their lung capacities and improving their vital signs. Improved balance, coordination, rhythm, timing, dexterity and general kinesthetic awareness are additional bonuses.

There are many reasons people exercise. The following is a list of some basic objectives, and where you can look to find out how one can use rebound exercise to reach those objectives:

	Read Chapters:
Maintain Health	VI, VII, IX, X, XIV
Increase work efficiency	VI, VII, VIII, X
Control weight	VI, X, XIV
Improve body symmetry	VI, VII, X, XI

Avoid disease	VI, IX
Reduce the effects of aging	VI, VII, VIII, IX, XI
Help correct physical defects	XI, XII, XIII
Improve skills and flexibility	VIII, XII, XIII, XIV
Build muscle, bulk and strength	VII, VIII

Rebound exercise can be achieved by using any piece of equipment that makes it possible to efficiently use the forces of acceleration, deceleration, and gravity without the shock and trauma of hitting a hard surface. The term "rebounder" is used in this text to identify any piece of equipment that can be used for rebound exercise. A list of equipment would include, but not be limited to:

trampoline — designed for tricks, considered dangerous.

rebounder — convenient, ideal, economical.

diving board — inconvenient, designed for dives, could be dangerous.

pogo stick — balance necessary, usually limited to those under 120 lbs.

spring board supported at both ends, used by visual therapists.

bed or couch — convenient, usually frowned upon by parents

branch or limb — hard to find, but fun when found.

Because we are concerned with the most efficient, effective, convenient form of exercise, we should concern ourselves with the best piece of equipment the one that was exclusively designed for rebound exercise . . . the rebounder. The following exercises have been identified as having specific benefits. We have labeled each by its benefit.

1. HEALTH EXERCISE

In the center of the re-bounder, move up and down by using your toes and your calf muscles. Your feet should not even leave the mat.

Bonnie Carter

Low Bounce

This is a good warm-up exercise. It is also good for re-lieving tension and improving circulation. Read Chapters VI, VII, IX, XII, XIII

2. AEROBIC EXERCISE

In the center of the rebounder, start a walking, jogging, or running motion. Lift your knees high in front of you. Do not wait for the rebounder to bounce your leg up — run at your own speed.

Randy Earl

Jogging Motion

The faster the motion and the higher the knees rise, the greater the aerobic demand. Hold on to a door frame or touch a wall if balance is a concern.

3. STRENGTH EXERCISE

In the middle of the re-bounder, use your toes and calves and bend your knees to bounce off the mat from 4 to 10 inches vertically so that you land in the center again.

Wendie Carter, 13

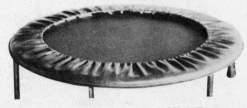

High Bounce

Read Chapters VII, VIII, IX. Hold a door frame or touch a wall if balance is a concern.

Other useful bounces:

Al Carter

Photographs by
Stephen Brady

4. TWIST

In the middle of the re-bounder, bounce so that the hips and legs turn to the left and the chest and shoulders turn to the right. On the next bounce turn the hips and legs to the right and the chest and shoulders to the left. On the next bounce, reverse again.

Read Chapter VII, XIV

5. DANCE

Turn on your style of dance music, get on the rebounder and "do it to it".

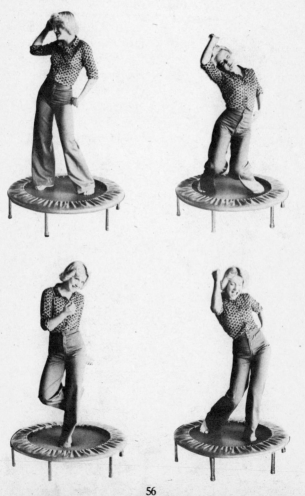

6. SLALOM (preparation for skiing)

With your feet parallel to the right of center and your toes pointing ahead and to the left, bounce and land so that your feet are parallel to the left of center and your toes are pointing ahead and to the right. Your knees and hips should be bent slightly. All of the action is below the hips so that the body remains virtually motionless and facing straight ahead (it is not as easy as it looks, but then neither is skiing).

7. HIGH KICK STEP

In the center of the rebounder, while landing on left foot, kick the right out straight in front of you, then land on the right foot and kick the left out straight in front of you. Do this for a few minutes and you have steam coming out your eyeballs!

This is an advanced move and should be tried carefully.

8. SITTING

While sitting in the middle of the rebounder, start bouncing by moving your shoulders and arms up and down. Read Chapters VIII, IX, XIV

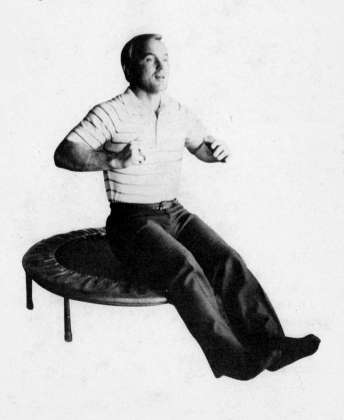

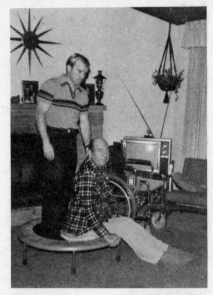

9. SITTING WITH ASSISTANCE

While sitting in the middle of the rebounder, have another person bounce on the rebounder behind you. Read Chapters VIII, IX, XIV

Read pages 162-166

Norman Nielson
(see p. 160)

10. WHEEL CHAIR REBOUNDING

Sitting in a chair next to the rebounder, place feet in the middle of the rebounder while another person is bouncing. Read Chapter XIV

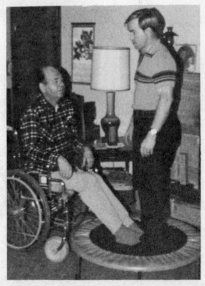

11. V BOUNCE

Sitting in the middle of the rebounder, lift your legs to a 45º angle while your back is at a 45º angle. Using the motion of your arms, try bouncing without touching the rebounder with your hands. Read Chapter VIII.

After interviewing many people who are rebounding every day, we have come to the conclusion that distance, height, and time are not as important as consistency. Rebounding five times a day is better than three times a day. Three times a day is better than one, and one time a day is better than no time at all. The following are suggestions to help you enjoy rebounding.

1. Select a definite place in the house or office. Call it the rebounding place — whether it is in front of your television, in your front room, recreation room, bedroom, or by your sauna or pool.

2. Make sure the rebounder is immediately available to everyone in the family, day or night, whenever they have the urge to rebound.

3. The most important time to rebound is within the first 3 to 5 minutes after you get out of bed. This will assist you in waking up, increase your cardiovascular efficiency, improve your lymphatic circulation, and act as a stimulus to cause all of the cells in your body to burn more calories throughout the day and be more efficient. Many people using the rebounder in this manner claim that they save as much as an hour a day because they are more alert and more energetic. This also helps eliminate the need for coffee, cigarettes and other stimulants often used for waking up.

4. If you are concerned about weight control, try rebounding 3 to 5 minutes at least 20 to 30 minutes before meal time and then allow your body to tell you how hungry you really are. Select a good nutritious diet that you have had previous success with, and stick with it.

5. Increase your rebounding only when you are ready. To train, it is not necessary to strain or to be in pain.

6. Give yourself variety. Some exercisers have a polka record that they call their rebounding music. Dr.

Henry Savage, M.D., rebounds while watching the news, or "Good Morning, America."

7. Try exercising during commercials of an exciting television movie, or turn on your radio and disco on the rebounder.

8. Do not strain or compete against the clock or against other people. Rebound as long as you enjoy it. Stop when you don't.

9. Involve the entire family in rebound exercise from beginning toddlers to grandma and grandpa who use walkers to get around. It may be necessary to connect a bar chest-high on a wall for those concerned about balance, equilibrium, or shakiness. Often, within a few weeks, this bar is no longer necessary.

At first, rebounding is not unlike opening a can of concentrated orange juice and trying to drink it straight from the can. Rebound exercise is concentrated exercise because three separate, potent, and previously unemployed forces are now being used all at once. Even seasoned athletes are amazed at how much exercise they get with so little time and effort.

If you are not exercising now and you begin to rebound, a word of caution is in order. Rebound for 30 seconds to a minute; get off and monitor your body. An hour later, get on again and go for another 30 seconds to a minute. If you do not have any ill effects, then increase your time to 2 minutes each time with at least a half hour in between; continue to increase until you find your threshold of limitation.

The objective of a good healthy exercise is to find your threshold of physical limitation and begin pushing it back systematically, consistently.

Each of us has our own peculiar physical limitations, and each limitation has its own threshold. Proper identification of one's own threshold is necessary for good physical development.

Common thresholds have been identified among people who rebound. We have compiled a few of them. It is important that you exercise to them, not through them. This list is incomplete because each has his own limitations.

1. **Headache** — most common among people who have not exercised. When headache stops wait half hour and rebound again. Usually the headaches disappear within a week because headache threshold has been pushed back resulting in fewer headaches.

2. **Leg Cramps** — most common among people who stand all day on hard surface. When legs cramp, get off rebounder and wait half an hour, then rebound again. Improvement within two or three days should occur.

3. **Panting** — most common among shallow breathers. Should notice improvement in two or three days.

4. **Excessive Increased Heart Rate** — most common among overweight people — especially those over 35 years old. Check with your doctor. Request ECG and stress tests to find any medical reasons why it would be dangerous to exercise vigorously.

As you approach each threshold, we suggest that you mark the approximate time on a calendar so that you can watch the improvement. Personal growth in fitness is extremely gratifying.

Here is a caution for the seasoned athlete who feels that rebounding is too easy. It is so efficient that you should not be surprised if you are sore the next morning should you overdo it.

Recent studies indicate that fewer than 20% of the people who start an exercise program using the accepted conventional programs such as jogging, cycling, jump rope, tennis, racketball, etc. are involved in the same

	6 a.m. (½ hr. before breakfast)	11:30 a.m. (½ hr. before lunch)	5:30 p.m. (½ hr. before dinner)	Daily Min. Totals
1st wk.	1 min. health 1 min. aerobic	1 min. health 2 min. aerobic	1 min. health 2 min. strength	
5 days/wk.	2 min. total	3 min. total	3 min. total	8 min./day 40 min./wk.
2nd wk.	2 min. strength 2 min. health	1 min. health 3 min. aerobic	1 min. health 3 min. strength	
5 days/wk.	4 min. total	4 min. total	4 min. total	12 min./day 60 min./wk.
3rd wk.	1 min. health 2 min. aerobic 2 min. strength 1 min. health	1 min. health 3 min. aerobic 1 min. health	1 min. health 4 min. strength 1 min. health	
5 days/wk.	6 min. total	5 min. total	6 min. total	17 min./day 85 min./wk.
4th wk.	2 min. health 3 min. aerobic 3 min. strength 1 min. health	2 min. health 4 min. aerobic 1 min. health	2 min. health 4 min. strength 4 min. aerobic 1 min. health	
5 days/wk.	9 min. total	7 min. total	11 min. total	27 min./day 135 min./wk.
5th wk.	2 min. health 5 min. aerobic 4 min. strength 1 min. health	2 min. health 4 min. aerobic 3 min. strength 1 min. health	2 min. health 5 min. aerobic 4 min. strength 1 min. health	
5 days/wk.	12 min. total	10 min. total	12 min. total	34 total/day 170 min./wk.

program a year later; whereas 80% or more of those who become involved in rebound exercise are still enjoying it a year later. This indicates that rebounding is convenient and the results are satisfying.

I have made an effort not to recommend an exercise program for anyone. Exercise is so individual that it would be unfair to many to reduce their horizons to a piece of paper. I would like to share with you an example of an exercise program that has worked for others, nevertheless. (Page 65)

The person who followed the above dropped from 210 lbs. to 180 lbs. in four weeks. His resting pulse dropped from 90 to 75 beats per minute. He reduced his blood pressure by 15 points and his cholesterol count by 25. Naturally, he used a diet that had worked for him before; but this time it worked more than three times as fast!

The best exercise schedule is your own schedule; one that you will start and continue. Why don't you sit down right now and draw one up for yourself. You'll be healthier and happier for it!

The rebounder's unique construction permits the body, through muscular contractions and bouncing motion to experience the forces of gravity, acceleration, and deceleration simultaneously. Because the human body cannot distinguish between acceleration, deceleration or gravity, it identifies all as increased gravitational pull. Each cell immediately works to adjust to the environmental pressure change created by the three forces. Each cell automatically works to strengthen its walls by a buildup of cellular protein. The rhythmic, vertical bounce reinforces the cells' initial neurological request for more cellular building material. Because this combination of forces is being applied to every cell in the body at once, each cell individually becomes stronger, and collectively strengthen the entire body.

Chapter VI
Rebounding Exercise
and the Lymphatics

"Rebounding is the best way to circulate the lymphatics. If the lymphatic system is circulating properly, it is practically impossible to get sick," I heard Dr. C. Samuel West, D.N., say in one of his health lectures. Well, now, what is the lymphatic system? Where is it? And, what does it do?

I had studied physiology in school, but the only thing that stuck with me about the lymphatic system was that any time I get sick the lymph nodes under my arms or in my groin swell up and hurt. If the lymphatic system is so important, why don't we know more about it? I didn't even know what it looked like. My research took me to numerous books and authorities. It's amazing what the general public **doesn't** know about how to keep well.

Are you aware that nearly 60% of an average person's total body weight is water? That one-third of the body fluid is extra cellular — meaning that it is on the outside of the cells? Like many other people, I just assumed that most body fluid was blood.

I was aware that man was made up of "muscle and blood, skin and bones, a mind that's weak, and a back that's strong." Nobody talks about lymph fluid. Since approximately 12% of the body fluid is blood, and 62% of the fluid is inside the cells, that means that 36% of the body fluid is lymph. There is 3 times more lymph fluid in the body than there is blood! ₈

Lymph fluid is that clear fluid that surrounds all cells. It is the cells' environment. The lymph is water, nutrients on the way to the cells, and waste byproducts excreted from the cells during nuclear reaction. Just as the air around us is in motion, so also is the lymph fluid around the cells. It is refreshing to receive a fresh breeze in a stuffy, polluted room; so also are our cells able to function better with fresh lymph that is filled with proper concentration of oxygen, glucose, different electrolytes, amino acids, protein, fatty substances, carbohydrates, and hormonal chemicals. When these replace the waste products of the cells, the toxins, poisons and trash that build up around inactive cells, we are healthier.

One of my questions was, "If the lymph fluid is the environment of the cell, and the lymph is in constant motion, what causes the lymph to circulate?" I knew that the blood is pumped through the arteries, lungs, capillaries and veins by the heart. I had seen pictures of the heart. I could feel it beat inside me, but where is the lymph pump? In searching for the answer I found that the "lymphatic system" had several nicknames, depending on the background of the person describing it. The most descriptive ones are: **"The Auxiliary Circulating System," "The Garbage Collector of the Body," "The Vacuum Cleaning System Within,"** and most recently, **"The Immune System."** Each one of these nicknames is very descriptive for a particular property of the lymphatic system.

"The Auxiliary Circulating System." We accept the cardiovascular system as the primary circulating system; rightly so because the heart starts beating before we are born and continues until we die. The cardiovascular system is complete with arteries carrying the blood to the capillaries, which, in turn, provide oxygen and nutrients to the fluid surrounding the cells — the lymph fluid —

and take the carbon dioxide and waste products from the lymph. The capillaries then deliver the blood to the veins, which, in turn, deliver the blood back to the heart after being filtered by the kidneys and lungs. Most everyone from the fourth grade on up understands the general cardiovascular function. But how many of us can describe the lymphatic system? **"The Auxiliary Circulating System"** is one of tubes whose cell walls are only one cell thick. They reach nearly every part of the body, and where the tubes don't reach there are minute passages where lymph can flow. The tubes start at the Lymphatic

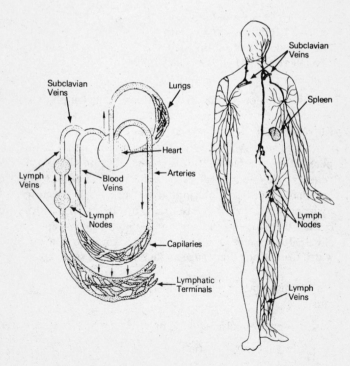

Terminals, which are located in the fingertips, toes, and other extremities of the body. The Terminal Lymphatics are very porous so that lymph fluid around the cells can flow into them.

The lymphatic tubes, for the most part, can be found next to the veins and arteries, and are located throughout the entire body; they connect the lymph nodes together and go through the spleen for filtration and finally emptying into the bloodstream at the subclavian veins behind the collar bone. [9]

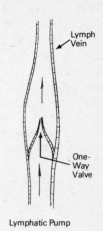

Lymphatic Pump

Okay, so now we have a description of the lymphatics. Where is the lymphatic pump? The lymph tubes are filled with millions of one-way valves like the veins in the cardiovascular system. In fact, there are far more valves per inch in the lymphatics than there are in the blood veins. These one-way valves are collectively known as the lymphatic pump. The lymphatics work on a pressure hydraulic system. Pressure built up below the valve causes it to open. Pressure above the valve keeps it closed. Increase in pressure causes the lymph to flow upward. Conditions that cause an increase in pressure are:

1. muscular activity — flexing and relaxing muscles,

2. changes in atmospheric pressure, and

3. change in gravitational pull.

Any decrease in pressure causes the lymph to move

sluggish. Conditions that cause a decrease in lymph flow are:

1. muscular inactivity — sleeping or resting too long, or convalescence, and

2. blockage of the Lymphatic Terminals by the oversized protein molecule.

It is easy to see why the Lymphatics System is called, by many, **"The Auxiliary Circulating System."**

"The Garbage Collector of the Body." Cellular activity gives off waste products into the lymph. Chemicals, which we unknowingly take into our body because of the additives in food that we cannot digest, many times find their way around the cells in the form of toxins, poisons, and extra-cellular trash. The lymphatics have the responsibility of pulling out the waste, toxins, poisons, trash, and excess protein from around the cellular tissue spaces. The more efficient the lymphatic system, the better it can do its job collecting garbage.

"The Vacuum Cleaning System Within." A vacuum cleaner creates a vacuum at the end of the hose causing air, dirt, and dust to rush into and fill the vacuum. The activity of millions of one-way valves causes a vacuum at the lymphatic terminals. The lymph fluid, filled with toxins, waste, excess protein, and dead cellular particles, is sucked into the lymph tubes to be filtered by the spleen and the lymph nodes. Recent research indicates a negative pressure in the interstitial spaces around the cells from -2 to as much as -10mm below the outside atmospheric pressure. It has also been determined that an efficient lymphatic system will keep the inside pressure a negative 6 at the end of the terminals. A body with a negative 6 lymphatic pressure will be a healthy body — toned and tight. However, like a vacuum cleaner, something too big would clog up the hose. The lymphatics can also be clogged. The major culprit is the huge protein molecule because it is more than five times larger than other molecules of the body. A major function of the lymphatics is to provide a passageway for the large protein molecule to get back into the blood stream. It is so big that it can just barely slip through the pores in the capillary membrane from the bloodstream into the lymph fluid around the cells; but it can't get back into the bloodstream through the capillaries. This agrees with information contained in *Medical Physiology*, by Arthur C. Guyton, M.D., Professor and Chairman of the Department of Physiology and Biophysics, University of Mississippi School of Medicine. He notes, ". . . the absence of any route other than the lymphatics through which trapped protein can return to the circulatory system. If trapped protein were not continually removed, the dynamics of the capillaries would become so abnormal within only a few hours that life could no longer continue."

The September 1973 issue of Scientific American contained an article on the lymphatics entitled, **"The Immune System"** by Niels Kaj Jerne. He shows how this diffused organ has the assignment of monitoring the identity of the human body. The lymphocytes and antibody molecules have the ability to recognize the difference between molecules of the body and foreign molecules. If the molecule is supposed to be part of the body, it is able to pass unmolested. If it is foreign or a mutant cell, it is identified and marked for destruction. The lymphatic system has the capability of ingesting and digesting foreign particles and building an immunity against future invasions of like foreign substances.

Now we come to an all important question: "How is the best way to circulate the lymphatics?" Answers:

1. Vigorous muscular exercise **will** cause an increase in circulation. A person's lymphatic circulation while running as fast as he can for 100 yards has been recorded

as much as ten times over his resting lymphatic circulation. [10]

2. Rebound Exercise has been found the most efficient method of lymphatic circulation stimulation because it yields the greatest change in pressure for the least muscular effort. When rebounding, the body is subjected to a change in velocity and direction twice with each jump. Each full bounce provides approximately two G's and a minimum of no G's. At the bottom of the bounce all the one-way valves are closed because of the pressure above them. At the top of the bounce the valves are open, allowing the lymph to flow up as the body starts down. Every valve opens at the same time, allowing the upward flow of lymph. At the bottom of the bounce, forcing all of the cells together squeezes the toxins, poisons, and trash out from around the cellular tissue spaces, making it possible for the lymphatics to vacuum them up and cleanse the body.

Eunice, age 83, was 90% bedridden. She always felt tired, drained, and useless to her family. Her daughter, Marion, brought a rebounder into her home. With a little coaxing, Eunice sat down on the rebounder while Bud, her spry 79 year old husband, proceeded to bounce behind her. This took place several times a day. Four days later, Eunice was up puttering around the kitchen, rinsing the dishes and wiping off counter tops. She no longer had to sit on the rebounder. She was standing, bouncing several times a day. Within eight days, Eunice was laughing and working around the kitchen, sweeping the floors, joking with her husband, and enjoying life again.

Basically, then, if the lymphatics function properly, we are healthy. If the lymph circulates improperly, we are sick.

The Health Bounce described in Chapter V on page 52 is all that is necessary for improving the health of

73

most people. Just a few minutes three to five times a day will do it.

By the end of the day, Helen's feet and legs were so swollen that, should she take off her shoes under her secretarial desk, she couldn't get them back on. Her legs ached — she could hardly wait to get home to sit down and get her feet up. Her feet were cold and blue from 2 o'clock on, every day. Bill heard about the rebounder from a presentation at his Kiwanis Club, and thought it might help his back; so he brought one home. Helen's first experience was exhilarating. She enjoyed the floating sensation and the tingling when she finished rebounding; but she was really excited four days later when she realized her trip home on the bus had not been a painful one. The circulation in her lower extremities improved so much that Bill no longer complained of cold feet in bed at night; and Helen was thrilled to no end one day when she got on the bathroom scale and found that she had lost over 12 pounds! She hadn't felt hunger pains, so her diet was much easier to stick with. She also noticed that her frequent headaches were no longer present! Bill dropped his chiropractic visits from one a week to one a month— then none at all. And he found that when he went from the second to the fourth floor in his office building, he no longer huffed and puffed as he used to.

I just received a letter from Bill and Helen Matson of Portland, Oregon and would like to share it with you:

"Dear Mr. Carter,

"I suppose I was as skeptical as anybody else when you began your presentation upon that small round trampoline. Twenty-five minutes later when you finished, I was thinking to myself, 'This is silly, but everything he said was logical.'

"Mr. Carter, I must admit I was desperate and I considered rebound exercise as 'any port in a storm.' I seldom write letters to speakers who make a presentation at our Kiwanis Club, but this time I want to thank you for the marvelous physical and emotional change that has taken place in our family.

"I have lost 52 pounds, my wife has lost 38. We arise every morning energetic and enthused with the prospects of the future because it is so much better than the past. Both Helen and I have tried almost every diet and fad and exercise program written, but this is the first time we have found something that is so fun, convenient and works — I mean **really works!"**

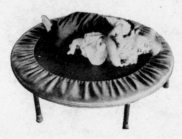

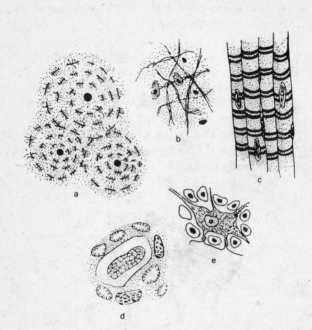

Histological sections of several tissues of the body, showing structural characteristics of different types of cells: (a) bone, (b) connective tissue, (c) muscle, (d) kidney and (e) nerve."

Chapter VII
Rebounding — A
Cellular Exercise

The basic living unit of the body is the cell. Each organ is actually a community of many different cells held together by intercellular supporting structures. Each cell is especially designed to perform its own special duty or specific function. The preceeding page illustrates five different types of tissues demonstrating different types of cells.

Although cells differ because of their structure and responsibilities, all have certain basic characteristics. Each requires nutrition for maintenance of life, and all use almost identical nutrients. All cells use oxygen as a catalyst to burn carbohydrates, fat, or protein. The general mechanisms for changing nutrients to energy are basically the same in all cells. The cells also deliver waste products of the chemical reaction into the surrounding fluids. Almost all cells have the ability to reproduce; and whenever cells of a particular type are destroyed, for one cause or another, the remaining cells of this type divide again and again until the appropriate number is replenished. Almost all cells respond to stimulation or exercise. They become stronger through increased stimulation, and they atrophy through lack of stimulation. Fluid outside the cells is known as extra cellular fluid. The extra-cellular fluid is comprised of nutrients needed by the cells and toxins and waste material excreted from the cells during the nuclear reaction. Extra-cellular fluid is in constant motion; therefore, all cells live in practically the same environment. Cells automatically live, reproduce, and adjust to their environment as long as proper concentrations of oxygen, glucose, different electrolytes, amino acids and fatty substances are available in the internal environment.

About one-third of the body fluid is extra-cellular — two-thirds is inside the trillions of cells that make up the body. A basic difference between the extra-cellular and intra-cellular fluids is that intra-cellular fluid almost always contains large amounts of potassium, magnesium, and phosphate instead of the sodium and chloride found in extra-cellular fluid.

Another essential difference between the fluids lies not in their nutrients or the excretory products, but in their electrolytes. Special mechanisms for transporting ions through cell walls maintain this difference. They develop a negative charge on the inside of the cellular membrane and a positive charge on the outside of the cellular membrane. This negative charge inside the cells makes it possible for cells to react to their environment electronically. Electrical stimuli permit a muscle to contract or relax. The stronger the stimulation, the greater the number of cells that become involved because of greater immediate imbalance of the electrical field at the cell membrane.

Incredibly, the cell is an intelligent entity in itself. It has within its walls the complete blueprint of the entire body. This blueprint is made possible by the combination of the chemical substances that make up the cell and is known as DNA (Deoxyribonucleic Acid). Although every cell in the body owns its own copy of the blueprint, it only reads that part of the blueprint that has something to do with its particular function. For example, a liver cell, once it becomes a liver cell, will always remain a liver cell. A skin cell will always be a skin cell, and a bone cell will always be a bone cell. The heart cell contracts rhythmically even if it is by itself, and when it contacts another heart cell, the two beat in unison continuously throughout their lives.

Red blood cells, the most abundant of all the body's cells, are adept at transporting oxygen from the lungs to the tissues. Their function and responsibility make it necessary that they be able to move around through the cardiovascular system without attachments. Red blood cells make up about 25% of all the body's cells. [12]

Obviously, I have merely touched the surface of cell physiology. But I believe it is enough to demonstrate how rebound exercise affects the environment of each cell individually, and therefore, collectively affect tissue, muscle, and bone.

Because every cell in the body has the ability to automatically adjust to its own environment, any change in the environment would stimulate that cell or group of cells. The cell is made strong by the amount and type of stimulation it receives. Most of the mechanical stimulation put on a cell comes from three sources: (a) atmospheric pressure, or environmental pressure; and (b) the gravitational pull of the earth; (c) muscular activity — called work. The greater the stimulation or pressure applied to the cell, the stronger it becomes because it constantly attempts to adjust to its environment.

The body's strength results from the overall strength of trillions of cells. They depend on the efficiency of the circulatory system. Just as the cell automatically adjusts to an environment, the human body also makes the same adjustmment. Strength and tone, then, depend on the overall demand made on cells and the health of the environment in which they live.

Cells become stronger to the point of rupture. As long as the stimulation, or pressure, is below the rupture threshold, the cell continually builds a stronger cell wall membrane to resist greater stimulation. This is evident when we are subjected to heavy manual labor. Our muscles become "hard as rocks" in a short time; but when some of the cells are stressed beyond the point of rupture, they are destroyed. We look at our blistered hands or feet and see the destroyed cells. As we continue to work, blisters are replaced by thick, tough calluses. Our cells have automatically adjusted to their new environment. If a person sits around and doesn't stress his cells, he becomes weak and flabby. The term "hard as nails" is used to describe the body of a vigorous, active athlete, or construction worker.

Rebound exercise is a method of stimulating every cell of the body simultaneously by increasing the G force applied to every cell. We do that by vertically adding the forces of acceleration and deceleration to the ever-present gravitational pull. Every cell in the body then begins to automatically adjust to the new environment.

For most healthy people, all cells are stressed well below the threshold rupture while rebounding so that rebound exercise is a healthy exercise for the entire body. However, injured cells, new cellular formations, aged cells, and cells weakened because of disuse have a very low rupture threshold. Hence, some elderly or extremely inactive people suffer from swelling or pain in their weaker parts while rebounding. This does not mean, however, that rebound exercise is not good for them. It merely means they should rebound with a gentler bounce — how gentle is determined by how weak their cells are. By gradually rebounding harder and longer they will have pushed back their rupture threshold to the point that they no longer have to worry about hurting something with the least amount of exercise.

Any change in an exercise program should be approached with caution; even more so with rebound exercise. Remember, we are tapping three sources of energy that we haven't considered using before. Therefore, we are working with an unknown result. We do not know how great an impact rebounding has on the human body. What we do know is that the reports are close to miraculous!

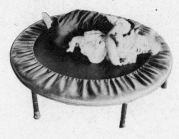

Chapter VIII
Rebound to Muscular Strength and Physical Fitness

The human body is a magnificent machine of levers. Each lever is controlled by two or more muscles of various design. Each muscle is designed specifically to do a particular type of work under very different and definite neurological commands. The more than 650 different muscles of the human body can be classified architecturally at least a dozen different ways, but once again, we are not going to talk about the differences of the muscles. We want to talk about their similarities.

Movement in response to an environmental change is one of the fundamental properties of animal cytoplasm. Leukocytes, a single cell, for example, have the ability to move away from an irritant by pulling in the cytoplasm (the cell fluid) at one point on its surface and flowing out or extending the cytoplasm at another point. The leukocyte, thus, is able to shorten the distance between two points or lengthen or extend its cell wall in another direction.

In multicellular organisms, certain cells, called muscle cells, become highly specialized for contraction and expansion. They are characteristically spindle shaped and are grouped in bundles to form a microscopic mass attached at each end and called a muscle. Muscles may be defined as organs that move parts of the body by shortening the distance between their attachments.

The three varieties of muscle tissues in the human body are usually described as (a) voluntary, or skeletal muscle, (b) involuntary, or smooth muscle, and (c) cardiac, or heart muscle.

Voluntary, or skeletal muscles, are usually the muscles we think of because these are what we use for locomotion. These are the muscles controlled by our thoughts and desired actions. When we think of developing a stronger physical body or comparing physiques, these are the muscles that receive our attention.

The involuntary, or smooth muscles, receive very little notice because they go about their business moving food through the digestive system, controlling vital organs, controlling the blood pressure in the arteries, and monitoring our body functions while we are awake or asleep.

The cardiac, or heart muscle, is one with the unique ability to pulsate or rhythmically contract from the moment it is identified as a heart muscle in the fetus until the body dies.[13]

The general concept of muscular development taught in school today is that it is necessary that a muscle be put through its full range of motion under stress in order to strengthen it. Weight lifters and health spas accept this concept because they are able to measure the strength increase by using that form of exercise.

Most exercise programs are designed to exercise specific groups of muscles. Push ups stress the extenders of the arms and chest. Pull ups stress the flexors of the arms and chest. Sit ups stress the abdomen and quadriceps.

Man has developed a sophisticated method of stressing all the striated or skeletal muscles by using different amounts of weight combining them with certain leverages and angles, and multiplying the effect on the body by specified repetitions of the same movement. Weight lifting has proved its value through the experiences of many of our athletes who participate in body building. The problem is that most exercise programs have been developed by athletes for athletes.

Although most of us have some hidden desire to be like Charles Atlas or Bruce Jenner, we recognize the improbability and are willing to settle for some exercise program that will merely help us endure to the end.

We turn to the experts and ask for a good exercise program to keep us healthy, and we are introduced to the exercise program used by the Royal Canadian Airforce, or to one used by our Astronauts. They work for those willing to pay the price in both time and effort.

So, the problem is that we have been convinced that the only way to develop strength in a muscle is to put it through a full range of motion with specific exercises.

If that were so, then a new baby would not only have to know the names of the more than 650 different muscles of the body, but also their locations, and the exercises necessary to work them. If these exercises were not carried out religiously by the baby, the muscles would atrophy by disuse. So you see, there must be another way to develop strength; a more natural way.

A muscle is a community of cells banded together to accomplish specific work. Like cells, muscles automatically adjust to the demand made on them from their environmental stimulation. Up to now we have accepted the method of stimulating our muscles by demanding that they contract through neurological requests from our mind. By repeating the stress stimulation, the cells request more calcium and protein and other building materials to develop stronger cell walls. The combined cellular strength of many cells results in stronger muscle.

Doctors, coaches and physiotherapists accept that

the formula for muscular strength is controlled stress X repetition. We have completely overlooked the fact that the very reason our skeletal muscles exist is to make it possible for us to move our frame around in the gravitational environment. Therefore, gravity is the greatest single stress influence on every muscle. Whereas work and exercise are available only periodically throughout the day, gravity is constantly present. If we were able to increase the gravitational pull of the earth by 10%, all muscles the world over would begin to increase in strength by 10%. Change the G force, and the environment has been drastically altered. Add the forces of acceleration and deceleration to gravity, and the cells of the muscles react to the increased G force. Do it over and over again, and all the muscles the body over will get stronger.

A few months ago, Dr. John D. Brown, D.C., of Redmond, Washington presented his family with a rebounder. His wife and all four boys enjoyed the convenience of exercising in their family room whenever they felt like it. Two of the four boys, Ron, 14, and Rob, 15, were in a weight training program at school. According to their weight charts on the coaches bulletin board both boys were increasing in strength by approximately 2½% a month as expected. Thirty days after they had started rebounding at home they both registered a 22% increase in strength, and followed the next thirty days with another 20% increase! The only change in their activities was their use of a rebounder. Every cell will adjust to an increase in G force if subjected to it repeatedly.

At eight years old, after being on the trampoline since he was three, Darren, my son, decided to see how many sit-ups he could do. He had never tried it before, but he was bored and needed something to do. I agreed to hold his ankles down, figuring he would do well to do 75 sit ups without stopping. He stopped at 429! I was amazed! However, he made two mistakes. One, he stopped simply because he was bored. Two, he did them in the front room with his twelve year old sister, Wendie, watching. Sibling rivalry being what it is, Wendie wasn't about to let her younger brother beat her in anything if she could help it. I held her ankles down. She stopped at 476 sit-ups! Why did she stop? Because she beat Darren. I still don't know how many sit ups either Darren or Wendie can do. Their only exercise has been regular rebound exercise on the trampoline.

A muscle need not be put through its full range of motion to strengthen it; to train it, yes, but to strengthen it, no. I have never lifted weights in my life; but in 10 years as an amateur wrestler through high school and college (Oklahoma State University) I never met an opponent in my weight class that I felt was stronger. My 24 years as a trampolinist has more than kept me in shape.

Dr. Alexander Leaf M.D. points out in his book, *Youth in Old Age,* that the difference between a mechanical device and our bodies is that a bicycle or an automobile can only deteriorate from wear and tear; but we improve with usage as long as we are in good health and the activity is not too violent. Our bodies respond positively to challenge. Strength, he says, is from development and enlargement of the individual muscle cell rather than increased numbers of cells.

1. Muscles, then, are communities of cells with one main responsibility — to contract upon demand thereby moving a bone or organ.
2. Muscles get their strength from the combined total strength of the individual cells.
3. To strengthen a muscle, the cells of that muscle have to be strengthened individually.
4. Each individual cell is an entity unto itself

capable of living, dying, multiplying, communicating, and adjusting to environmental stimuli.

5. Cells are banded together into muscles to accomplish work impossible for them to do individually.

6. The main purpose of a skeletal muscle is to move part of the frame against gravity.

7. Muscular strength is a measure of the ability of a group of cells to contract when stimulated.

Many people mistake the terms "strength" and "fitness". Now that we have discussed strength, let's look at fitness.

A muscle may be strong, but if the necessary oxygen and nutrients are not available to the cell when demand is made on the cell, or if there are too many toxins, wastes, and poisons around the cell, making it impossible to function properly, it will become fatigued. It will not be physically able to keep up with the demands. A body wherein these conditions prevail is considered "out of shape".

Physical fitness is a measure of circulation efficiency. Increase circulation efficiency of the body fluids — the lymphatics and the blood stream that services the cells — and the body is then considered physically fit; the muscles are able to continue the same work longer, without fatigue.

Rebounding not only increases the strength of each muscle by increasing the G force repeatedly, but also increases the fitness of the muscle by improving lymphatic and blood circulation in the muscle.

Dr. Leaf went through several stages of thinking regarding the fitness, health, and longevity of persons living more than 100 years. His studies led him to the Caucusus in Russia, Vilcabamba in Equador, and Hunza in Pakistan, where he met, photographed, and examined the world's oldest people. The remarkable things about those people — dozens of them over 100 years old — are their extraordinary health, high spirits, and full, productive lives. Searching for their secret, Dr. Leaf examined them — listened to their hearts, took their blood pressure and watched them dance — even saw them bathe in ice cold mountain streams. He interviewed them about their daily lives, their hopes and fears, and their histories.

He speculated that their remoteness protected these people from infectious diseases. He found, however, that most varieties of infectious disease were present.

He considered the possibility that their remoteness fostered intermarriage, which brought about a dominance of genes favorable to long life. But, the common belief is that there are no genes for longevity — only genes that decrease susceptibility to fatal diseases. Inbreeding generally causes degeneration of the stock.

Dr. Leaf analyzed the influence of altitudes between 2,000 and 6,000 feet; but altitude showed minimal effect. He considered the purity of the air and lack of pollution. He finally concluded that the high level of physical fitness needed to survive on steep terrain was very important. To get through a normal day's work required great physical exertion. No one sat around at a desk or rode to and from work. To get from one community to another required great physical exertion. Walking to the fields from their dwellings left Dr. Leaf huffing and puffing; but even the oldest natives negotiated these steep slopes agilely. "Retirement" or "desk jobs" were not in their vocabulary. Walking up and down hills required cardiovascular and lymphatic fitness.

Studying their heart and lung functions, using the modern sophisticated techniques, Dr. Leaf found that many of these people had cardiovascular diseases; but the illnesses were apparently silent and not accompanied by the usual symptoms simply because each cell was able individually to withstand normally lethal stresses of heart attack.

Physical fitness, then, is just as important as strength. Usually, when an athlete thinks of strength exercises, he thinks of weight lifting. When he wants fitness, running comes to mind. Now, he can get both by rebounding. The higher the bounce of the rebounder, the greater the G force at the bottom of the bounce. The greater the G force, the stronger the cells become. A jogging or running motion on a rebounder increases body fluid circulation for better fitness. What could be simpler or more convenient?

We are frequently asked to compare rebound exercise to jogging or jumping or whatever. But because there are so many elements to each exercise, it's impossible to make any meaningful general comparison.

We have established what we feel is a fair and equitable point system for 21 activities. We have researched already published physiology for this comparison. Since there is little agreement among experts as to caloric burn and other values (because everyone is different) we feel we should say that this chart has been produced for comparison purposes only and your own experiences may vary (sounds like an EPA gasoline disclaimer heard on TV, doesn't it?).

The formula for establishing a total point value for the various activities is as follows:

1. 1/6 of the calorie consumption per hour of a 154 pound person.
2. Each activity has been classified in the following six categories.
   A. muscular development
   B. general endurance
   C. flexibility
   D. balance and coordination
   E. safety
   F. convenience

They have been given a value based on whether

ACTIVITIES EVALUATION CHART

5 Points = Poor   10 Points = Good   15 Points = Excellent

Activity	Calories Used Per Hour			Muscular Development	General Endurance	Flexibility	Balance	Safety	Convenience	Frequency	Frequency Points	Total Points
	114 lb.	154 lb.	194 lb.									
Rebound-sprint	1260	1440	1710	10	15	15	15	15	15	3/day	105	430
Jumping rope	590	750	930	5	10	5	15	5	15	1/day	35	215
Running	590	750	930	10	15	5	10	5	15	3/wk	15	200
Skiing	630	810	990	10	10	10	15	5	5	occ	5	195
Swimming-butterfly	780	840	900	10	15	15	15	10	5	1/wk	5	215
Rebound-strength	870	1050	1230	15	15	15	15	15	15	5/day	175	440
Basketball	510	630	750	10	15	10	15	5	10	3/wk	15	185
Bicycling-15 mph	510	690	810	10	15	5	10	10	15	1/day	35	210
Swimming-back stroke	480	600	600	15	15	15	5	10	5	1/wk	5	175
Weight lifting	540	660	780	15	5	15	5	5	10	3/wk	15	170
Football	480	600	720	10	10	10	10	5	5	1/wk	5	155
Karate	420	540	660	10	5	10	10	5	5	3/wk	15	150
Mountain climbing	480	600	720	10	15	10	10	10	5	occ	5	165
Rebound-jogging	480	600	720	15	15	15	10	15	15	5/day	175	365
Bicycling-10 mph	360	420	480	10	15	5	5	10	15	1/day	35	170
Calisthenics	300	360	420	10	5	10	5	15	15	1/day	35	155
Dancing	270	330	390	5	10	5	10	10	15	1/wk	5	120
Table tennis	270	330	390	5	10	5	10	10	10	1/day	35	140
Walking-outside	300	360	420	5	10	5	5	15	15	1/day	35	150
Rebound-health	90	150	210	10	10	15	15	15	15	5/day	175	280
Walking-indoor	90	150	210	5	10	5	5	15	15	5/day	175	255

it is classified as excellent, good or poor, in that classification. Excellent receives 15 points, good — 10, and poor receives 5 points.

G. Each activity has been calculated by the recommended frequency per week and has been given 5 points for each time it is recommended per week.

Example: one day a week has a value of 35 points, 5x7; one time a week is only 5 points and 5 times a day would be 175 points, 5 times a day x 7 times a week x 5 points.

Using this same formula you should be able to calculate for yourself the total points for any activity you're interested in and compare it to the published activities.

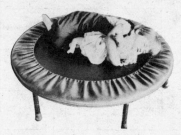

Chapter IX
A Vital Exercise for Vital Organs

Now that we know what builds muscle, we can apply that same simple information to build stronger, more efficient vital organs. How? We get on a rebounder and gently move up and down approximately 100 times a minute for three to five minutes three to five times a day.

The human body is a magnificent creation! Various of its organs are responsible for controlling the homeostatic condition of the environment for the individual cell. Many hundreds of control mechanisms are necessary to control the very important conditions such as arterial pressure, oxygen concentration in the tissue fluids, carbon dioxide concentration, and the rates of individual chemical reactions in the individual cells. The purpose of exercise is to control the environment, or, let's say, to stimulate control of the cells' environment. Just as we are concerned about the energy and freedom to do what we want in our own environment, every cell in the body is likewise. Each cell has to be free to do its own thing without bothering the function of other systems. Each organ must work in harmony with each other. Just as the police department must work in harmony with the fire department. The sanitation department is as necessary to our environment as are our hospitals. Nevertheless, all control systems of the body have certain characteristics in common.

Most of the body's major control systems and organs operate by means of reflexes. One element of a system acts as a receptor, a second acts as a transmitter, and a third as an effector.

In nervous reflexes, the sensory organs are receptors; the nerves — including the pathways through the central nervous system — are transmitters, and the organs at the end of the motor nerves, muscles of the skeletal system, muscles of the blood vessels, cardiac muscle, gland and other structures, are effectors.

Hormonal reflexes work in much the same way. In the glucose regulatory mechanism, the receptor is the Islets of Langerhans of the pancreas, which secrete insulin in response to the increase in a glucose concentration. The transmitter is the insulin, and the effectors are the membranes of all body cells that are stimulated by the insulin to increase their rates of glucose transport from the extracellular fluids to the intracellular fluids. For the most part, the body's control mechanisms and organs involve either nervous or hormonal reflexes.

Most body organs function by reacting to opposition to their neutral position. For example, in the regulation of carbon dioxide, concentration in the extracellular fluid causes an increase in pulmonary ventilation; this, in turn, causes decrease in carbon dioxide concentration. Conversely, if the carbon dioxide concentration falls too low, opposition to the homeostatic or neutral position results and causes the concentration of carbon dioxide to rise. Concentration of glucose is regulated this way along with arterial pressure. Therefore, if the extracellular fluid becomes imbalanced in any way because of too much or too little of anything, a control system, or a group of organs, initiates a series of changes that cause an opposite reaction. This always keeps the environment of the cell near a certain concentration, thus, maintaining homeostasis.[14]

Two of the main stimuli that cause negative feedback to body control mechanisms are change in atmospheric pressure, and change in the gravitational pull of the earth. Therefore, the stimulation of rapid vertical movement of the body on a rebound unit causes all vital organs to work harder at controlling the body's environment.

Increased stimulation from rebounding a few minutes three or four times a day, has prompted many people to claim that the rebounder cured many physical problems. Some, therefore, would like to label the rebounder a miracle machine. But the rebounder is not the miracle machine — the body is. The rebounder merely assists the body's many organs to function more efficiently.

CAUTION: We should issue a word of caution here. Some believe that if a little exercise is good, much is even better. Others believe they are strong enough to withstand greater physical exertion than they really can. And some of us don't know really what is good or bad for us. In a recent article from *The Reader's Digest*, May 1978, we read of abnormal presence of protein, red blood cells, and other substances in the urine that indicate a serious kidney disease known as "joggers kidney." It is not really a disease but a condition caused by prolonged exercise on a hard surface. A specialist in sports medicine, Dr. Robert Johnson of Knox College in Gailsburg, Illinois, estimates that as many as 10 million joggers exhibit signs of joggers kidney. That's about 40% of all joggers in the nation!

All exercises should be properly studied and evaluated. And if one attitude should dominate others, it would have to be conservativeness. Do not over exert yourself; build your endurance slowly. Rebound exercise is so easy that many beginners rebound too long the first time and suffer for it the next day.

It is quite common for a lady to get on the rebounder, bounce up and down three or four times, and immediately feel she has to relieve her bladder. She will come back, get on the rebounder, and in fewer than a dozen bounces, return to the rest room. This is unnerving; and immediately she says to herself,

"I cannot use that because of the continual bathroom trips."

What she doesn't realize is that the internal organs have been accustomed to the environment of 1 G, or just the ordinary gravitational pull. Any vigorous activity would cause the same sensation. When one increases the G force, the increased pressure creates the need for release because the bladder is weak and is easily activated by a slight increase in internal pressure. The person accustomed to vigorous activity, a trampolinist for example, does not have this problem. All internal organs, because they are made up of cells that individually can adjust to new environment, will adjust or become stronger with increased and repeated stimulation. The bladder is an organ that will immediately indicate a weakness; but all organs in the body have adjusted to the same G force as the bladder. Within one, two, or three weeks of rebounding, people who experienced weak bladder problems no longer have those problems. This is an indication that not only the bladder has become stronger by enrivonmental adjustment, but that all other internal organs, cell by cell, have strengthened. Rebound exercise not only strengthens all muscles and the entire skeletal system, it also strengthens all vital organs, cell by cell.

The largest organ in the body is the skin. Right after a mother has her baby, one of her immediate concerns is to get back to her girlish figure. Her doctor may suggest some form of exercise, such as sit-ups. So, for the next sixty days, she faithfully performs her sit-ups and other recommended exercises. She has developed a very strong abdomen and other related muscles, but she still has the flab of the abdomen recently stretched out of position. If this young mother had spent the same time and effort rebounding as doing sit-ups, she would not only have strengthened her abdomen, but would also have virtually eliminated the excess skin tissue; even the skin is exercised through rebound exercise! A team of Finnish researchers has found that those people who exercise have a thicker, more flexible skin. The researchers also theorize that exercise may slow down the aging of skin. *(British Journal of Dermatology,* August, 1978.) The skin, then, tones and tightens, and the mother is back to her girlish figure.

Most exercise programs suggest how a person can strengthen, tone, and tighten the voluntary muscles of the body. But show me a published exercise program that is designed to strengthen the spleen, kidney, pancreas, and all other vital organs. Keep in mind that just as a chain is only as strong as its weakest link, a man is only as strong as his weakest vital organ.

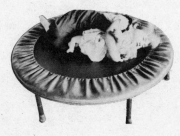

Chapter X
Aerobics is Necessary, but . . .

In the middle 60s, the works of Dr. Kenneth Cooper began to show up on the news stands in doctor's offices and coaches' training rooms. The medical term *Aerobics* was popularized and soon people all over the nation began to talk about earning aerobic points, a measure of oxygen consumption. His book has been accepted by the United States Air Force, the United States Navy, the Royal Canadian Air Force, and many medical clinics and sports medicine clinics. It has been read by everyone serious about exercise.

"Aerobics" is the term used to define the function of cells that need oxygen to burn foodstuffs to create energy. All of our cells need oxygen to create energy from the food we eat, so they are aerobic. Any activity, including sleeping, needs energy. So we need oxygen. The body is able to store food, but it is unable to store oxygen. But because we live in an atmosphere of oxygen, we are able to replenish our supply just by expanding our lungs. The problem is not that of supply — it is that of delivery.

Cardiovascular efficiency, then, is the underlying message of Dr. Cooper's book. Through his studies he has found that the greater the activity of the heart, arms, and legs, the greater the pumping action of the blood to get the oxygen to all parts of the body. Walking, jogging, swimming, cycling, running, and stationary running have become known as the aerobic exercises because they have been shown to deliver greater amounts of oxygen to all cells more efficiently.

Because the entire cardiovascular system has the ability to automatically adjust to environmental stresses, vigorous activity has been known to actually develop new circulation to the muscles. New capillaries are able to carry more blood to the body's muscles with each beat. This new circulation is called collateral circulation.

Increased activity stimulates an increase in the manufacturing of red blood cells. The blood contains more hemoglobin and has greater oxygen grabbing capacity. The result is that a significantly greater amount of oxygen can be carried per quart of blood.

The heart is a muscle that, if increased in strength under controlled environmental stress, improves cardiac output. The heart can thus either do more work with each beat, or the same work with fewer beats. Therefore, the heart rate drops after using a good aerobic exercise for a few weeks. While the average American has a resting pulse rate in the neighborhood of 75, trampolinists and runners are notorious for having pulse rates as low as 45. (My resting pulse rate has been recorded as 39.) This means that an athlete with an efficient heart saves about fifteen million heart beats a year!

The increased demands on the body's arteries improves their elasticity. To transport blood effectively under differing needs, the arteries must contract their inside diameters on command. Our arteries have a tendency to harden and become less elastic as we age, making such contractions difficult. Aerobic exercise reverses this trend causing arteries to become more rather than less elastic, easier to contract.

The efficient heart is more able to cope with sudden uncontrolled body stresses such as illness or accidents. Because of improved circulation, recovery time from body damage is shorter, resistance to fatigue, stress, and pain is greater.

It is little wonder that Dr. Cooper's books made such an impact on his readers. Many scanned his books and decided that aerobics was the answer. Millions began running. Others started jogging.

Today, over 25 million people are jogging because they misread the leading books on aerobics and running.

Dr. Cooper warns of starting too aggressively or being ill-equipped.

Dr. George Sheehan, M.D., Cardiologist and confirmed runner, author of *Running and Living*, states that if you run, you have to be willing to pay the price of injuries. He claims that some of us shouldn't even attempt running because our bodies are not capable of coping with the shock and trauma of continually hitting a hard surface.

Dr. Roger H. Michael, Chief of Orthopedic Surgery at Union Memorial Hospital in Baltimore, states that jogging causes more injuries than any other sport. These injuries include muscle strains, pulled ligaments, and joint inflammation.

As many as ten million, it is estimated, are suffering from "joggers kidney", a condition of over exercise.

Who needs aerobic exercise? We all do. Who needs the pain and suffering normally expected with most aerobic exercises? "Not I," we all say. Then, what is the answer?

Allow me to answer in this way: Cooper's premise is that the answer is oxygen circulation to the cells. Granted, oxygen is necessary; but perhaps he was too close to the real answer to recognize it. Perhaps the real answer is efficient body fluid circulation to the cells. You see, any activity that would cause increased oxygen circulation would also cause increased fluid circulation. Therefore, as aerobics was studied, all of the benefits appeared to be because of efficient oxygen consumption; when, in fact, many of the benefits of the activity were a combination of better lymphatic circulation, better delivery of nutrients by the blood, more efficient oxygen utilization from the lungs, and better elimination and digestion because of more efficient body fluid circulation.

Maximum cardiovascular efficiency can be achieved by rebounding aerobically five four-minute periods each day. Any longer than that is not going to improve heart efficiency noticeably.

It makes no difference how much oxygen is available to cells if the right nutrients are not there. Even if oxygen and foodstuffs are readily available, with too many toxins, poisons, or trash in the lymph fluid surrounding the cells and hampering proper cellular function, good health would not be likely.

The body can't possibly have an overly efficient fluid circulation system. Efficient fluid circulation is synonymous with physical fitness.

Body fluid circulation is the answer. What aids in body fluid circulation? Certainly we would have to accept all "aerobic" exercises because they also activate the natural fluid pumps of the body. But are all the aerobic exercises best for the body? Not if 50% or more of the participants are injured while participating.

The natural body fluid pumps are activated by any change in pressure, whether internal or atmospheric, and by any change in the G force. The most effective way to activate the natural body fluid pumps is by rebounding vertically.

Our concentrating on better circulation will cause us to breathe deeper automatically, thereby getting all of the aerobics necessary.

Your challenge is to study the concepts of this book and either prove, disprove, or use these concepts for better health.

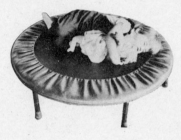

Chapter XI
A Safe Answer to Jogging

Although bones are more rigid than either muscle tissues or vital organs, the cells that make up the skeletal system are also alive, and, because they are, they too are subject to environmental adjustment.

Dr. Alexander Leaf, mentioned in Ch. VIII in connection with his studies of aged people in Russia, Equador, and Pakistan, had much to say about skeletal systems. He found that although our elderly people often suffer from osteoporosis, or bones weakening from becoming more porous, the centurians he studied seldom broke bones when they fell. He pointed out that, with activity, their bones remained mineralized, dense, and strong. With inactivity, bones become weak, porous, and fragile. Bones are constantly eliminating old and building new cells. If we have remained active, the new cells become stronger. The greater the activity, the stronger and more dense bone becomes.

Because the gravitational pull has such a great influence on the environment of every body cell, an increase in the G force causes the skeletal system to become heavier and stronger. A decrease in the G force causes it to become weaker.

After two weeks of weightlessness in outer space, our astronauts lost up to fifteen percent of the bone mass from their skeletal systems. Their bones were adjusting to the new environment. Dr. Chestnut, University of

Washington, pointed out that women beyond menopause as well as astronauts suffer from osteoporosis. Is it possible that rebound exercise can arrest and even reverse osteoporosis? Let's analyze it.

Suppose every cell in the body can automatically adjust to its environment. Suppose gravity has a direct influence on the environment of every cell in the body. Suppose you can increase the gravitational pull by controlling acceleration and deceleration vertically. And the astronauts actually did lose fifteen percent of their bone mass because of weightlessness for fourteen days in outer space. Doesn't it seem entirely possible, then, that by rebounding enough to increase the G force three or four times a day, the bones would stop getting weaker? And, by adjusting to an increase in the G force, might they not even grow stronger?

In Dr. Ken Cooper's books on aerobics, he indicates that jogging is one of the best exercises for increasing heart efficiency. He also points out the importance of a person's wearing proper shoes and going through the necessary warm-up procedures to keep from injuring the skeletal system.

Dr. George Shehan, M.D., whom we cited earlier as a cardiologist and confirmed long distance runner, indicates that stress and injury while running is inevitable. He explains the problem as a structural, almost architectural one — not a medical one. Weak muscles along the front of the lower body sooner or later tear, pull, strain, sprain, or stress fracture.

Dr. James D. Key of Dallas is one of the many medical doctors who calls this situation the "over use syndrome." The over use syndrome is multiplying rapidly in the thirty to fifty age group of amateur athletes who run daily because they want cardiovascular fitness. Among a group of surveyed athletes, forced to stop their activity for as long as two weeks because of pain, the knee was the principal problem. Following closely were problems involving inflammation of the Achilles' tendon, shin splints, pain in the arch of the foot, ankle injuries, fractures of the foot, pains in the muscles of the leg calves, hips, thighs, and pain in major bones of the leg. The lower back is often referred to as the "soft underbelly of the jogger" because of jogging's toll in injuries to the lower back.

A Chicago physician, Dr. Gordon Falknor, identifies traumatics and tendonitis of the Achilles' tendon, just above its attachment to the heel bone, as "joggers ankle." He agrees that terrific pounding from jogging on concrete, blacktop, or other hard surfaces leads to the inevitable breakdown of tissue.

Dr. J.E. Schmidt, M.D., in his article, *Jogging Can Kill You,* is even more adamant about jogging as an exercise. He states that jogging is one of the most wasteful and hazardous forms of exercise known — it takes more from the body than it gives back.

It endangers the lower back, or the sacroiliac joint, he states; jogging adds a ballistic impact of the lower spine each time the foot of a jogger hits the ground. It is not unlike splitting a log with a sledge hammer. The discs of the back, under excessive pressure, often burst, expelling the contents. Medically, this is known as a herniated disc. We call it a slipped disc.

Dr. James White of the University of California in San Diego, in *World Wide Report,* February 1978, noted this: Several university staff members, who stopped their previous fitness programs, have recorded significant weight losses after a few weeks of rebound exercise workouts. According to Dr. White, people with lower back pain or minor knee, hip, or ankle injuries can rebound because minimal or no additional pain occurs while exercising. Several U.C.S.D. faculty and staff members who had begun walking, bicycling, or swimming programs for fitness, but who had to quit due to increased pain, can and do exercise vigorously by rebounding. Dr. White stated that when you run or exercise on a solid surface, a certain amount of force from the impact of the heel striking the ground is sent throughout the body. On a rebounder, the mat is so yielding that the impact force is absorbed over a longer period. Dr. White has been studying rebound exercise in his laboratory in San Diego for more than a year. [15]

Dr. Gideon Ariel of Amhurst, Massachusetts, a biomechanical scientist, has studied the effects of rebound exercise for more than two years. He states that if you take the bad out of jogging — the shock or trauma of hitting a hard surface — and leave the good things in, you have an optimal system of exercise. Rebound exercise accomplishes this, precisely.

Chapter XII
And the Eyes of the Blind Shall See

Four out of ten grade school children in the United States are visually handicapped. Their grades and achievement in school suffer from it. Many of these visually handicapped students, along with their parents and teachers, are unaware that they have a visual problem; unfortunately they were endowed with good clear 20/20 sight.[16]

"I have perfect 20/20 vision," I heard my son say when he came home from school one day. Like millions of students all across the nation, he was given the very same eye test I received dozens of times while I was going to school; these were the same charts that were devised in 1863 for determining if one could see with both eyes at twenty feet what one should see at twenty feet. The average near-sighted child has been handed spectacles similar to those worn in Benjamin Franklin's day.[17]

Dr. Arnold Sherman, associate professor of optometry, New York State University, tested 50 children who had scored 20/20. Seventy-five percent of them had vision perception problems. Ninety percent had poor eye/hand coordination. The eye chart tests commonly used in schools only test the visual acuity and sharpness. They do not test indirect field of vision, eye muscle action, speed of seeing, effort needed to see, or ability to see clearly at a near point.

Old ideas die hard; but there is quite an effort being exerted to correct the old concept about "perfect vision".

First, there is no such thing as "perfect vision." Surprised? I was. I have always had the mistaken idea that visual capabilities were sort of inherited. If mom and dad were near-sighted, all of the children were going to wear glasses. If mom and dad had perfect vision, then the children didn't have to worry about glasses.

That's wrong.

Research tells us that visual capabilities are as individual as our thumb prints. My good vision may not be the same as someone else's good vision. The fact that vision is different things to different people is sometimes hard to understand until we're really introduced to what vision is.

Dr. G.N. Getman, O.D., one of the foremost visual therapists in the nation, and author of "How to Develop Your Child's Intelligence," makes the statement: "Good vision is the **learned** ability to gain the most information from the fewest clues."

Just as I was, most people are under the impression that we are born with vision. That is not so. Just as we are born with arms and legs which we have to learn how to use through trial, error, and exercise, we are also born with eyes, which we have to learn how to use properly.

Vision is a function of the brain. As a child develops, the eyes pick up information and send it to the brain for classification. If the visual clue is familiar, it has meaning. If not, then it is filed away for future reference in the memory bank. Any visual clue that has meaning starts a chain of events that forms a single visual process. Failure in any single step in this process can create problems. A child learns visual skills or abilities just as he learns to walk and talk. Unfortunately, he doesn't have the opportunity to mimic his parents and siblings as he does in learning other skills. We can watch a child learn to roll over, sit up, crawl, stand, walk, run, etc., and assist the learning procedure; but learning to see is a process that generally goes on without assistance, many times without concerned and informed awareness.

A child who is learning vision:

1. must first learn where he is. Identify his arms and legs and control their direction and movement.
2. must learn to co-ordinate his left half with his right half.
3. must learn where he is in relation to other visually observable objects.
4. must memorize sizes, shapes, depths, distances, speeds, locations.
5. must learn to function in a gravitational environment.

The sight mechanism is quite complicated but, simply stated, works this way: To pick up a message both eyes must be pointed in the right direction and be focused for the right distance. The muscles that control focus and direction must work together. They must be perfectly balanced and make tiny adjustments hundreds of times a minute. The message is sent to the brain. Vision is based on experience, memory and reliability of the incoming information.

To learn, a child must have mastered all of the above. Problems begin when an incorrect message is received at the brain.

Disappointment, frustration, and failure in school are a few of the penalites that await the unsuspecting student who is visually unready to learn.

Some of the signs of poor vision in a student are observable behavioral patterns. The student:

confuses letters or words,
reverses letters or words,
skips or re-reads,
vocalizes when reading silently,
reads slowly,
uses his finger as a marker,
has poor reading comprehension,
covers or closes one eye,
moves his head excessively,
tilts his head to one side,
holds reading close,
holds his head close to the desk when reading,
frowns or squints,
rubs or blinks his eyes excessively,
writes or prints poorly,
tires easily,
is inattentive,
daydreams,
is aggressive,
is withdrawn,
has temper flare-ups,
cries frequently,
shows poor general body coordination,
rejects hand-eye activities,
must feel things to see them,
complains of headaches,
complains of blurred sight,
complains of eye discomfort,
has reddened eyes or red lids,
tears excessively,
has frequent sties on lids,
sees double,
confuses left/right direction repeatedly,
avoids all near centered tasks,

squirms, fidgets and is hyperactive,
suffers from car sickness,
makes errors in copying,
does little or no voluntary reading at home,
distorts his posture when reading or writing,
omits small words,
has short attention span,
daydreams in class,
displays clumsiness on the playground.

Naturally, any child or adult who suffers from any of the above visual problems is going to have more than his share of learning problems.

Most people are surprised to learn that vision can be improved with exercise. They assume that one is born with either good or bad eyes. The idea of improving eyesight through exercise can be traced to the Egyptians; yet we have been so convinced that we have no control over the condition of our eyes that we calmly accept gross disorder as simply . . . "that's the way things are."

I'm reminded of the story of the patient who had a slight head cold. He went to his doctor and said, "Can't you do something about my runny nose?" The doctor pulled out a clothes pin and attached it to his patient's swollen red nose and said, "Wear that the rest of your life and you won't have to worry about the sniffles again." We usually have our eyes checked when they are really bothering us. The optometrist verifies what we already know, fits us with glasses, and we wear that crutch the rest of our lives.

One rather interesting book on the subject of Sight without Glasses is authored by Dr. Marilyn B. Rosanes-Berrett, *Do You Really Need Glasses?* published by Hart Publishing Co., Inc. 1978. Her book, along with literature from The College of Optometrists in Vision Development, P.O. Box 285, Chula Vista, California 92012, and extensive communication with eye specialists all over the nation, has caused me to "open my eyes" about vision. I am convinced that as high as eighty percent of all people wearing glasses could eliminate their glasses if they found the right exercises and did them regularly.

I was surprised to learn that the shape of the eyeball changes under stress, pressure, exercise, nutritional deficiencies, illness, shock, or trauma. Although the eye is one shape one day, it may be a different shape the next.

Dr. William W. Bates, a New York opthalmologist, a graduate of Cornell and of the College of Physicians and Surgeons, while examining more than 30,000 eye patients a year, became increasingly disturbed by the difference between what he had been taught and what he was observing. He noticed that some of his patients could see better on some occasions than others. He noted that hyperopia (far-sightedness) and myopia (near-sightedness) would come and go on some of his patients. This led him to the conclusion that the eyeball must be able to change shape, and therefore, could be influenced by emotional stress, strain, and even exercise.[18]

In the 1920s, Dr. A.M. Skeffington developed an exercise program for eye treatment. Until that time, only prescription lenses had been used. His techniques forced the eye to be used in ways it had not been used before.

Research at the Gesell Institute of Child Development, The National Institute of Health, The Optometric Center of New York, Texas Association of Children with Learning Disabilities, and other research centers has advanced the concept that vision can be influenced by exercise.

The work of Dr. Hans Selye, the world's foremost authority on stress, showed that all living things — all parts of the body — have to adapt to prolonged stress or die. A muscle that is subjected to greater stress either strengthens or completely breaks down. All this is directed by a central intelligence center in the brain that receives information, analyzes it, and sends back commands. The eyes are no exception.[19]

The new idea that vision is improved by proper exercise is the reason for the Fellowship of College of Optometrists in Vision Development. A new science called Development Optometry combines the knowledge of psychology, neurology, child development. It and other related fields have given us a new concept of vision.

Our eyesight has a great deal to do with personality. If affects what we think and how we are. If we improve our visual skills we will improve the coordination of the entire body and mind. We expand the horizons of our own world ". . . and the eyes of the blind will see out of obscurity and out of darkness."

So, how do we exercise the eye? We can't do push-ups or leg lifts with muscles behind the eye that control the direction of the eye. We would even have a hard time telling which muscle or group of muscles needed exercise and which ones were functioning properly. Visual therapists have developed a number of exercises that have proven beneficial under specific circumstances. The list includes:

1. putting pegs into holes on a revolving turntable;
2. standing in front of a blackboard drawing circles with each hand at the same time;
3. looking through a gadget and tracing simple pictures;
4. playing with pieces of plastic triangles, rectangles and squares and putting them together to form different shapes.

5. standing on a teetering board while staring at a multi-colored revolving disc;
6. wearing thick training lenses to create an extra blur and trying to pick out at random letters on a ball swinging at the end of a cord;
7. pointing to numbers on a chart to the beat of a metronome.

Some of the above tasks may sound uncomplicated; but to a person with impaired vision, doing them is another matter.

Visual therapists all over the world report amazing new ideas about vision when a patient is willing to exercise the eyes. Some of their conclusions are:

1. Defective vision may be influenced by emotional strain. Relaxed and healthy, we see our best;
2. Stress can be relieved by exercise. Eyesight will improve when avoiding stress or strain, sometimes fast, sometimes slowly.
3. Growing older is inevitable. Farsightedness is not. With aging, we lose flexibility of muscles, but through proper exercise we can maintain that flexibility.
4. The eyeball is not fixed. Hyperopia and myopia (presbiopia and near-sightedness) are not permanent. It can be changed constantly subject to both positive and negative factors.
5. Eye glasses generally do more harm than good. They are intended to correct errors of refraction. Glasses make reading and seeing more comfortable, so it takes less effort to demand that the eyes perform satisfactorily. Dependency on the glasses is established, making them a crutch, which does not treat the underlying cause of the visual error.[20]

Please understand that I am not admonishing you to get rid of your eye specialists. That would be like telling a football team to get rid of its coach because the team does all the work and he just stands on the side, yelling. What I am saying is that your eyes are yours; and it is your responsibility to keep them healthy and demand what you expect of them. Most people who are obese, are so because they are willing to accept themselves as such. Likewise, most visual problems are accepted weaknesses. Chances are good that, should you decide to solve your visual problem, you will be able to eliminate your glasses. A good visual therapist will be happy to help you.

A fourth grader attending a class for the mentally retarded since kindergarten appeared to be heading for a future requiring the simplest vocational skills. A guidance counselor, who was aware of the visual advances, recommended the boy be given a complete visual examination. They found the student was unable to coordinate both eyes smoothly. The information being taken in was jumbled, causing severe perceptual and thought-organization problems. He began a visual therapy program involving weekly visits to an optometrist, exercising on a small trampoline, and excercises at home. A year later, he tested normal intelligence and was transferred to a regular class.

Where does rebound exercise fit into visual therapy? We get this information from the top visual therapists in the nation. Dr. G.N. Gettman, O.D., as an example, in his article, Use of Trampoline in the Developmental Visual Guidance, states that,

> "A trampoline, device for rebound tumbling, has usually been considered a gymnastic equipment, and too frequently, one of its real values has been overlooked . . . the trampoline provides opportunities for the acquisition of basic movement control, which is essential to coordination. Clinical and research studies of rebound exer-

cise indicate that the trampoline can provide experiences that influence a child's academic success. Many authorities recognize that a child's freedom to learn and his readiness for new learning experiences is dependent on his freedom and control of movement. This control movement must come from the visual mechanism because the eyes are the primary steering machinery for all movements. *The trampoline contributes more to the organization of visual perception than any other known device* ... these optometrists are recommending rebound tumbling for the improvement in the total visual and body control. It is not used solely for the building of muscle bulk and strength." (see page 176).

Dr. Gettman recognized that rebound exercise was excellent for building muscle bulk and creating strength. He went one step further and stated that, (a) the trampoline contributes more to the organization of visual perception than any other known device, (b) all children should use rebound exercise, (c) especially the clumsy child should use rebound exercise. He stopped just barely short of stating that rebound exercise is the most efficient, effective form of exercise yet devised by man; but then, he had not heard the revolutionary new concepts presented in this book: "gravity is the common denominator of all exercises," and "the greater the gravitational influence on the body, the stronger each muscle will become when overcoming that opposition."

The trampoline has been with us for more than 40 years, but very few people have considered it as a form of exercise. Very few have, that is, except for the visual therapists who have used the trampoline as a therapeutic exercise tool for at least 30 years.

It was a real pleasure to walk through the very

pleasant new office building of Drs. Stephen L. Jaffee, O.D., and Theodore S. Kadet, O.D., in Issaquah, Washington. It contains an observation room employing one-way glass. Parents or other interested parties can view the visual therapist and patient during optometric training. The visual therapy room is equipped with some of the latest instruments for development of better visual perception. I watched a visual therapist direct a young third-grader to a small three-by-six foot trampoline. It stood in a pit in the floor so that its surface was about floor level. This was not an experiment — it was part of the visual therapy. Most people are surprised when they hear that rebound exercise had been used for more than three decades to assist better visual efficiency.

Recently, I was asked to speak to a visual therapists meeting in Seattle. I explained to them that, while rebounding, every cell is impressed at the bottom of the bounce, while every cell in the body is weightless at the top of the bounce. The contrast between the G force at the bottom and the weightlessness at the top creates quite a dramatic impression on every cell in the body.

I explained to the visual therapists that the bottom of the bounce was the point of learning. Improved vision comes about when the millions of cells in the eyes and the muscles controlling the eyes are individually impressed to do a better job because of increased environmental stress. And because they already know their jobs, they begin to function properly. At the same time, the kidneys, gall bladder, pancreas, heart, lungs, and all other internal organs are receiving the same message. One of the visual therapists responded,

"I have been using a small trampoline in my practice for 20 years. Now I can see why rebounding improves the vision of our patients."

Several of the visual therapists in the Seattle area have been enthusiastically assisting me to develop a few exercises that will help improve your vision by using the rebounder at home under adult supervision. Here are some suggestions from that program:

General Rebound Visual Exercises:

1. Always use a comfortable, well lighted room. Distractions should be eliminated as much as possible.
2. Prepare the room with one bulletin board so that, while bouncing, the participant can look directly at the board on the wall. Charts for the board are included in Chapter XIII.

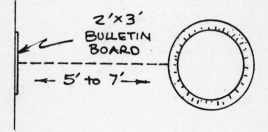

3. Do not wear your glasses while rebounding.
4. Rebound going through the basic exercises on pages 52-54. Many times the cause of poor vision is stress caused by worry, fatigue, anxiety, pressure or illness. Rebounding will eliminate many of the causes and poor vision will begin to improve automatically.
5. Using the health bounce look at various objects around the room — with both eyes, the left eye, then the right. Concentrate on seeing them clearly.
6. Focus on something on the floor far from you, then near.
7. Focus on something on the ceiling far from you, then near.
8. Look out the window and follow a moving object such as a dog, car or person. Concentrate on clarity.
9. Stop bouncing. Close your eyes and concentrate on what you have just seen. Think of seeing them clearly.
10. Open your eyes and look at the objects you were just thinking of.

11. Rebound with your eyes closed.

12. Caution: do not overdo these exercises. Stop before you fatigue your eyes.

13. Remember, your eyes have adjusted to the demands you have placed on them through years of use. It is important to be consistant and patient with your exercises.

14. These exercises can be done two to five times a day as long as there is plenty of rest time in between.

15. Should you follow the above exercises you will have exercised your entire being. The exciting tingling sensation throughout your body when you finish will verify the improved body fluid circulation.

Eye Exercises for Nearsightedness:

1. Warm up with some or all of the above exercises.

2. Attach a chart, similar to the one on page 131, at eye level while standing on the rebounder, to a bulletin board, the wall or door.

3. Place the rebounder at a distance away from the chart where the symbols become fuzzy.

4. Rebound concentrating on seeing the symbols clearly. Do this one to five minutes three to five times each day.

5. Keep the rebounder at that distance until you see the symbols clearly. When you do, move it 6 to 8 inches farther away and start over again.

6. The eyes adjust every day to internal and external stimulation. Don't be discouraged if you have to move the rebounder closer on some days. Most people see clearer in the middle of the day and while exercising. Eye exercises are not as effective just before bed time because the eyes are tired. Do your eye exercises when you feel good.

7. These exercises can be done two to five times a day for three to five minutes each time as long as there is plenty of rest in between.

Eye Exercises for Farsightedness:

1. Warm up by doing some or all of the general exercises.

2. If you are not able to focus within arms length, pin up bold print on a bulletin board and locate the rebounder as close as possible still being able to read the print.

3. Using a very low health bounce, concentrate on clarity

121

of the bold print. Close one eye, then the other, then use both. Move the rebounder closer as your ability to focus improves.

4. If you are able to read within arms length, use the general visual exercises above before sitting in a comfortable chair in a well lighted area in an upright position, preferably at a desk. Concentrate on bringing the reading material closer to your eyes and still be able to read. Do not fatigue your eyes. As soon as your eyes get tired, stop reading and rebound for a few minutes, then go back to your reading. This can be done several times in succession.

The suggested exercises in this chapter can be used by almost everyone who wants to improve their vision. However, they do not take the place of your glasses. They are possible ways of eliminating the need for glasses. Your eye specialist should be consulted should you question your visual capabilities. Some visual problems cannot be corrected by exercise, but most can be improved.

Suggestions for Visual Training for your children will be included in the next chapter. Many visual problems of our youth are simply a lack of educational training and can be eliminated by playing educational games on the rebounder under the guidance of an informed adult.

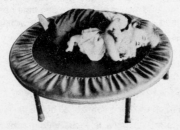

Chapter XIII
Startling Break-Through in Education

For the past thirty years, visual therapists have been using small trampolines to assist patients in developing better vision. Most people believe that vision is hereditary, and therefore unquestioningly accept their visual capabilities. Visual therapists have found that vision is a learned procedure and is subject to training. Through the experience of many optometrists and educators, the evidence is overwhelming that most students do not learn to see well enough by the time they start school. The teacher, the parent, and the child all fight a losing battle when the child's ability to see is poorly developed. As children learn to visualize, they learn to look and observe. They learn to see more in less time. They gain the visual ability to substitute symbols for experiences. They learn simple hand and finger manipulation as a visual activity, which, when properly applied, produces a good writer, a good reader, and a good speller. Because 80% of everything we learn comes through the eye, good visual training is vital throughout our education process.

Dr. Robert C. Pepper, O.D., Lake Oswego, Oregon, is very concerned about the multi-sensory approach to educational therapy programs. In the past, visual therapy has been mainly directed towards those children who have developed visual problems as the result of prolonged visual stress. Visual therapists are now concerned with the holistic approach of visual therapy.

123

The recent move to holistic medicine has brought visual therapists, psychiatrists, and special education instructors closer together in working with children who are educationally handicapped. Essentially they have found that:

1. Gross Motor Control is the ability to move the body where and when one wants to.
2. Eye-Hand Control is the ability to direct the hand with visual clues.
3. Eye Control is the ability to focus the eyes and identify objects correctly.
4. Visualization is the ability to remember objects, clues, and symbols, memorize things, and dream of past experiences and abstract concepts.
5. Visual-Auditory-Language relations is the ability to read, write, and describe what is seen or read.
6. Organization is the ability to interrelate all five of the above skills.

With the use of this book, parents will be able to be actively involved in the visual and educational training of their children the fun and easy way.

On the rebounder, rhythm and timing are essential to the student's learning activities; constant and steady rhythm must become adequate in neuromuscular coordination. Incorrect rhythm is noticed by the instructor immediately. Therefore, he has immediate student feedback as to whether the desired response is correct. Regardless of the participant's age, rebound exercise will help these aspects of his life:

balance
tactile and kinesthetic awareness
positive body image
coordination

spacial awareness
timing
rhythm
self-confidence
attention span
behavior
problem solving and positive learning skills
visualization/visual memory
voluntary muscle action
breathing habits
endurance
caloric burn
lymphatic circulation
self-esteem

Many psychiatrists notice better behavior, and instructors and educators notice better problem-solving and positive learning skills. They find that children who were formerly failing the first or second grade are now able to achieve A and B grades. Many of these improvements are brought about because the child has learned to visualize better. Visual therapists are now recommending rebound exercise to the psychiatrists and special education instructors because they see such phenomenal improvements.

Dr. G.N. Gettman, O.D., made the statement that trampolining provides opportunities for the acquisition of basic movement control, which is essential to coordination. Studies of rebound exercise indicate that the rebounder can provide experiences that influence a child's academic success. (See page 178)

Rebound exercise embodied in trampolining has been used in elementary schools, junior highs, and high schools to assist many children to develop better balance and coordination. I personally have seen many students change from introverts to extroverts through trampoline instruction. I have been called in to counselors' offices on several occasions and told by the counselor that the student's grade had improved so dramatically that I should continue whatever I was doing through trampolining.

There are many cases on file verifying such work of special education instructors with mentally, emotionally, socially, and physically slow or handicapped children through use of the trampoline to bring out dramatic improvements. Dr. Alfhild Akselsen of Texas has been successfully using rebound exercise for the slow student. Physical therapists, special education instructors, psychiatrists, and athletic coaches all appear to be converging on the same concept from different directions. That concept is that rebound exercise produces amazing physiological results.

In one of my lectures at Bellevue, Washington, November 29, 1977, I was explaining the theory that the bottom of the bounce was the point of education. Dr. Gideon Ariel was in the audience. He is one of the foremost biomechanical scientists in the nation and has done research with rebound exercise. Half way through my presentation, he stood up and walked to the back of the room. Immediately, I thought I had said something he didn't like. After my presentation, he came up to me and said,

"Al, you have just explained why the results of one of my laboratory tests turned out so positive."

He then excitedly proceeded to explain that he had studied a group of tennis players, each having at least five years experience playing tennis. Each was to hit a tennis ball through a thirty-inch hole in a 4 x 8 sheet of plywood at the other end of the tennis court. They were all instructed to use the forehand stroke. Half of them were on the tennis court practicing as usual. The other half attempted the same feat while bouncing on a rebound unit. From the final outcome of the test, Dr.

Gideon Ariel was able to conclude that testing results show a player using rebound exercise as a tennis teaching aid in practice drills improves his accuracy more than 100% over the players who didn't. His results were so amazing that rebound exercise received the endorsement of the United States Professional Tennis Association.

What an exciting breakthrough! Until this time rebound exercise was considered to be useful only to the physically or visually handicapped. But these students were college athletes! Their accuracy was improved by rebounding.

After rebounding for only 60 days George Janson, the Athletic Director of Tiffin University, dropped his golf score from 100 to the low 80s!

These and other exciting results of rebound education verify the theory that the bottom of the bounce is the point of learning.

A closer look at rebound education will help us understand the correlation between exercise and education.

Just as the common denominator of all exercises is opposition to the gravitational pull of the earth, so also, the common denominator of education is cellular stimulation and memorization.

We know that cells can be stimulated to memorization at least four ways:

(1) neurologically — an impulse through one of the five senses impresses the cells to necessary memorization;

(2) electrically — every cell reacts to an electrical imbalance causing muscles to move in cellular memory reinforcement;

(3) chemically — any imbalance in the chemical environment causes cells to react; and

(4) mechanically — by mechanically repeating

a movement we are able to memorize that movement. Many autistic children are assisted in learning to crawl when several assistants mechanically move the child's arms, legs and head to simulate the child's natural crawling motions.

Until recently it was thought that all of the intelligence of the human was in the brain. We are beginning to realize that, although thoughts and actions are coordinated in the brain, the actual learning procedure takes place in each one of the cells individually.

It is scientifically accepted that each individual cell is an entity unto itself capable of living, dying, procreating and adjusting to environmental stimulae. However, each cell owns a blueprint of the entire body of which it is a part. This blueprint is the DNA (deoxiriboneuclic acid). The blueprint is so complex that it is able to record every stimulation received by the cell throughout its entire lifetime. Each cell memorizes its own stimulation. Our memory is the sum of the response of each cell responding to a central demand.

Although each cell owns its own blueprint, it only reads that part of the blueprint that has something to do with its purpose. An eye cell is always an eye cell. A liver cell is always a liver cell. Hairy skin tissue grafted to another part of the same body will grow hair.

When we come to understand this concept it is easy to accept the fact that each cell knows its own responsibility. **We did not have to know how to function to be.** As a baby we did not have to study the eye to see, nor the ear to hear.

Our living causes cellular stimulation; and the fact that we function properly indicates that our cells have memorized the stimulation so that repeating a move is easier.

Education in part is organized cellular stimulation aimed at a desired coordinated result.

Therefore Exercise **is** Education.

Since each cell already knows its own function, any increased stimulation will cause the cell to memorize and function more efficiently.

Memory is a prerequisite to education. Before an organism can learn, it must be able to record or memorize an experience. Man is no exception. One learns slowly to drive a car; an executive secretary capable of typing over 100 words per minute must begin her first typing lesson.

My wife has won three national honors in piano. Today, she can sit at the piano with no music in front of her and play Bach's two part inventions or one of many other memorized pieces. Simultaneously, without missing a note, she can instruct my daughter, Wendie, in household chores. That talent is not accidental. It took years of practice. Every muscle and every nerve from the fingertips to the brain knows what it is supposed to do at a given response.

Neuromuscular coordination is a product of constant and steady rhythm and timing. This is equilibrium; the instant feedback that the body receives about its orientation in space from rebounding makes it possible for educators to say that no other motor skill activity is quite this precise. Hands, arms, head, eyes, body, and legs learn to work together to develop proper balance and coordination. Because the bottom of the bounce is the point of learning, the student's response at the bottom of the bounce would assist him to learn. Let's suppose that a child is having difficulty learning the alphabet. Clinical results show that bouncing on a rebounder aids memorization; while facing an alphabet chart hanging on the wall seven to ten feet away at eye level, a child asked to recite the next letter each time he lands on the rebound unit, would quickly be able to master the alphabet.

A properly trained special education teacher will recognize danger signals. Rolling of a student's eyes, the change in bounce, the reversal of arm movements, the repetition of the same number or form, tenseness of the body or fingers, or any variation of the relaxed, comfortable bouncing motion indicates a mis-motor match. It is a signal that the student is having trouble. Either the demand placed on him should be lowered, or the student should be encouraged to work out the problem.

Rebounding is convenient. Students should be encouraged to rebound several times a day rather than all at once; thus, developing the benefit of spaced repetition.

Mental attitude, attention span and physical fitness capabilities should be standards by which the time limit is placed for each activity or learning period.

Rebound education has been used primarily for special programs for the handicapped. It has also been successfully used to assist average students in learning such things as multiplication tables, spelling, geometric forms, and even biblical quotations. Each time rebound education was used, the students were able to comprehend and master the skill faster and with greater retention. Adults have been using rebounding to improve tennis and golfing scores. Professional athletic organizations have been using rebounding techniques to improve peripheral vision by demanding identification responses from charts attached to opposite walls while the athlete is rebounding and looking straight ahead. Professional skiers have improved their skiing techniques and endurance during the summer by rebounding. Several basketball teams have already improved their back board techniques under the net by rebounding on the sidelines on a rebounder.

After recently talking to a number of educators who

have been using rebound exercise, I became so enthused about rebounding techniques that I decided that I might benefit from rebound education. I had attempted, a number of times, to learn the piano from Bonnie in the past fifteen years. I understand my problem is not unfamiliar to music students — that is, being able to identify the position of the note of an octave on the piano keyboard, or identifying the name of the note in the base clef or the treble clef of written music without counting from middle C. When I arrived home, I immediately made a chart of the position of the eight notes in the octave and pinned it to the wall in front of me. Then I

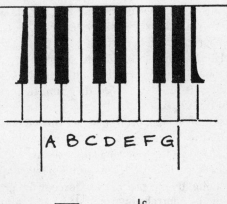

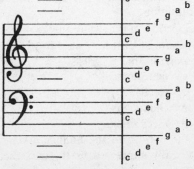

mounted the rebounder and for, 20 minutes, studied the chart making identification responses at the bottom of each bounce. Twenty minutes later, to my amazement, I had the positions of the notes on the keyboard memorized. I then took a chart of the treble clef and the bass clef and went once again to the rebounder. Twenty minutes later, I emerged from the bedroom a musician! I could read the position of the notes on written music and immediately play it on the piano. Both Bonnie and my mother-in-law, Velma Rogers (both are piano instructors), were as amazed as I with the results.

Since that time my family has been using the rebounder to memorize music, multiplications, and school assignments. We are even teaching 2½ year old Melynda the alphabet. I will draw a single letter on paper on the bulletin board and tell her what it is.

"Melynda, that's a 'B'." I will say. She then gets on the rebounder and every time she lands she recites, "B . . . B . . . B . . . B . . . " She then runs to an alphabet book and finds a 'B'.

The statement has been made in this chapter, "The bottom of the bounce is the point of learning." This theory is based on the following suppositions:

1. Every cell is an entity unto itself, capable of living, dying, procreating (except for nerve cells in the central nervous system) and adjusting to stimulation.
2. Memorization is a pre-requisite of learning.
3. There are at least four ways to stimulate a cell to memorization:
    a. neurologically
    b. electrically
    c. chemically
    d. mechanically
4. At the bottom of the bounce **every** cell is mechanically impressed by the increased 'G' force

caused by the combination of acceleration, deceleration and gravity.

5. Every cell records forever on its own DNA chain every environmental impression.

6. The demand to learn visually and the increased 'G' force impression is accepted as one stimulation because each cell cannot tell the difference.

7. Repetition of the 'G' force impression and the learning demand is reinforced at each bounce, requiring each cell to indelibly record the desired learning skill.

8. The balance, coordination, rhythm timing, etc. are outward manifestations of internal cellular education.

Now that we know what rebound education is and how it works, let's put it into practice. Depending on physical space available and what goals are established, here are three recommended teaching stations.

Teaching station I

Single bulletin board teaching station

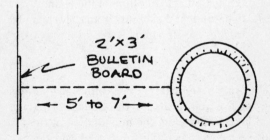

This teaching station is sufficient for most visual therapy and basic learning techniques. Counting, alphabet, colors, multiplication, phonics, spelling, reading, shapes, symbols.

Instructions: The student stands in the middle of the rebounder facing the bulletin board. Bounce so that feet just leave the mat. Recite at the bottom of the bounce, **NOT** while feet are in the air.

Example:

Chart A, alphabet

Step 1.   Teacher points to 'A'.
Student recites at bottom of bounce:
"A . . . A . . . A . . . A . . .

Step 2.   Teacher points to different letter each time.
Student recites at bottom of bounce.
"A . . . B . . . C . . . D . . . etc.

Step 3.   The student looks at the chart without the instructor's assistance and responds each time he bounces.

Step 4.   The student and the instructor recite the letter at the same time while the student is bouncing.

Step 5.   The student closes his eyes and visualizes the chart and responds.

Step 6.   The chart disappears from the wall, or is covered up, and a response from the student is requested at the bottom of the bounce.

Step 7.   The student dismounts from the rebounder and recites the alphabet.

The following charts are only suggestions for achieving different goals for the student. They are presented here to stimulate the imagination of the teacher. Create your own charts to fit your circumstances.

Chart A
Alphabet upper case

A	B	C	D	E	F
G	H	I	J	K	L
M	N	O	P	Q	R
S	T	U	V	W	X
Y	Z				

This chart is easiest to teach the alphabet.

It is also used for visual therapy because it is so easy to identify.

Charts B, C, D, are variations to demonstrate how one concept can be expanded.

Chart B
Alphabet - lower case

a	b	c	d	e	f	g	h	i	j
k	l	m	n	o	p	q	r	s	t
u	v	w	x	y	z				

Each letter one bounce

Chart C
Alphabet - lower case - backwards

z	y	x	w	v	u	t	s	r	q
p	o	n	m	l	k	j	i	h	g
f	e	d	c	b	a				

Each letter one bounce

Chart D
Vowels

a	e	i	o	u	a	e	i	o	u
u	u	e	i	i	o	a	e	u	o
e	e	a	o	o	a	i	a	u	u
o	a	o	a	i	u	u	u	i	i
u	i	e	i	e	e	a	e	o	u

1. d b g p q f t d b d b
2. g p g q f t d b d b d
3. b b d d f t d b g g b
4. g g d d f f p p q d b
5. n n u u n n u u n u n
6. p p q q p q p p p q q

Each line can be expanded into another chart.

Chart F
Spelling

bat	girl	cat	sat	rat	hat
find	lost	now	how	cow	bow
say	pay	lay	pray	play	day
pat	vat	fat	mat	etc......	

Each word — one bounce.

Chart G
Words Phonics

pic nic	pub lic	box top
of ten	up set	hab it
fab ric	pup pet	riv er
hot dog	sus pect	gal lon
vel vet	etc......	

Each box two bounces.

Charts H - J Color Identification

Chart H

RED	YELLOW	GREEN	PINK			
BLUE	BLACK	ORANGE	GREY	BROWN		
GREEN	RED	PINK	BLACK	PURPLE	BLUE	

Colors and words in each box

Chart I

RED	YELLOW	GREEN	PINK			
BLUE	BLACK	ORANGE	GREY	BROWN		
GREEN	RED	PINK	BLACK	PURPLE	BLUE	

Words only in each box

Chart J

Colors only in each box

139

Counting — Number Identification

1	2	3	4	5	6	7	8	9	10
11	12	13	14	15	16	17	18	19	20
21	22	23	24	25	26	27	28	29	30
31	32	33	34	35	36	37	38	39	40
41	42	43	44	45	46	47	48	49	50
51	52	53	54	55	56	57	58	59	60
61	62	63	64	65	66	67	68	69	70
71	72	73	74	75	76	77	78	79	80
81	82	83	84	85	86	87	88	89	90
91	92	93	94	95	96	97	98	99	100

Chart L
Mathematics-Form Identification

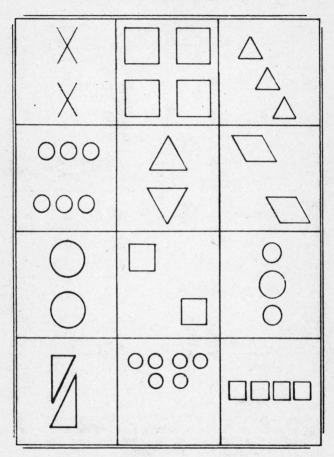

Student responses: 2 . . . 3 . . . 4 . . . 6 . . .
Triangle . . . circles . . . squares . . . crosses

Teaching Station 2

Four-bulletin board teaching station.

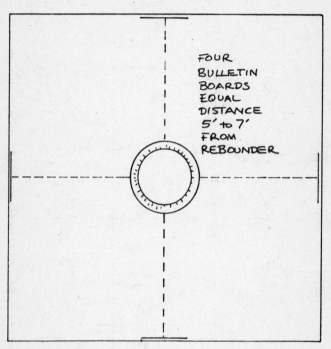

FOUR BULLETIN BOARDS EQUAL DISTANCE 5' to 7' FROM REBOUNDER

2'x3' bulletin boards

This station is useful for teaching **all** that can be taught with Teaching Station 1. It has been expanded to teach effectively the concepts of direction, size, right and left, time, front and back, opposites, choice, color. Develops balance, coordination.

Teaching Station 3

Four-bulletin board teaching station unequal distance.

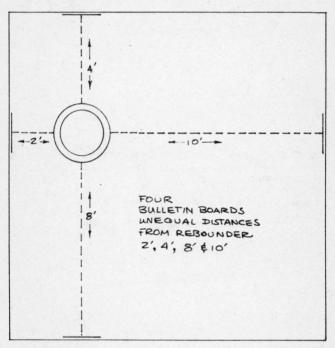

FOUR
BULLETIN BOARDS
UNEQUAL DISTANCES
FROM REBOUNDER
2', 4', 8' & 10'

2'x3' bulletin boards

Distances are unequal.

This station will be useful for teaching all of the above skills, adding depth perception to them. This is the most ideal setup for teaching both visual and educational skills to students of various visual capacities and educational needs.

Charts: Each chart is placed on different bulletin board.

Chart Sets M

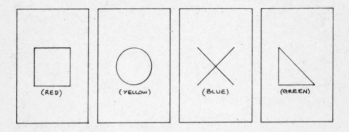

While the student is bouncing, the instructor calls a demand at the bottom of the bounce. The student faces that board on the next bounce. Instructor's demands could be:

1. Red . . . . . yellow . . . . . green . . . . . yellow, etc.
2. Left . . . . . right . . . . . right . . . . . left, etc.
3. Square . . . . . cross . . . . . circle . . . . . square, etc.

Chart Sets N

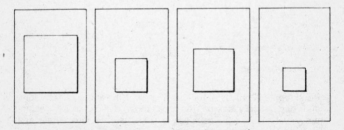

Instructor demands: Largest . . . . . smallest . . . . . larger, etc.

Student would face the proper board at the bottom of the bounce after turning in the air.

Chart Sets O
Time — Direction

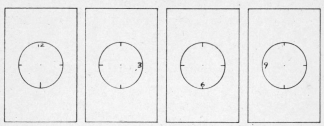

Instructor demands: Top .....bottom .....left .....right .....
noon .....3 .....9 .....1 .....5, etc.

Chart Sets P
Alphabet Direction

A	B	C	D
E	F	G	H
I	J	K	L
M	N	O	P
Q	R	S	T
U	V	W	X
Y	Z		

Instructor requests the alphabet. The student will be bouncing clockwise. By exchanging the second and fourth chart, the student will bounce counter clockwise while reciting.

Chart Sets Q
Mathematics

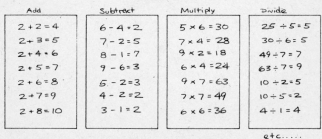

Add	Subtract	Multiply	Divide
2 + 2 = 4	6 – 4 = 2	5 × 6 = 30	25 ÷ 5 = 5
2 + 3 = 5	7 – 2 = 5	7 × 4 = 28	30 ÷ 6 = 5
2 + 4 = 6	8 – 1 = 7	9 × 2 = 18	49 ÷ 7 = 7
2 + 5 = 7	9 – 6 = 3	6 × 4 = 24	63 ÷ 7 = 9
2 + 6 = 8	5 – 2 = 3	9 × 7 = 63	10 ÷ 2 = 5
2 + 7 = 9	4 – 2 = 2	7 × 7 = 49	10 ÷ 5 = 2
2 + 8 = 10	3 – 1 = 2	6 × 6 = 36	4 ÷ 1 = 4

etc......

Each chart represents a series that can be expanded.

Chapter XIV
Success Stories

Testimonials from those who have observed or actually experienced the benefits of rebound exercise.

These stories and letters have been written in their own words. Very little editing has been done.

DOROTHY HOWARD

Seattle, Washington

There she is — over there carrying that small round trampoline. At 67 she's a spry young lady. Younger than three years ago when her doctors told her that she would soon be in a wheel chair because of her condition. That bleak news didn't slow her down. She had been living with her left leg three inches shorter than her right all of her life. At ten months, she had polio that impaired the normal growth of her left side. Through special effort she had learned to type using both hands, but her left foot remained cold and numb.

At 64, with the probability of a wheel chair in the near future, she was introduced to rebound exercise by Jerry Hinkle. She began rebounding religiously. In less than a month she noticed feeling in her left foot for the first time in 60 years. Her foot was no longer cold. After two months of rebounding she found that she had to learn to walk all over again because she was able to walk with her left heel down on the floor, something she had not been able to do all her life. Six months into rebounding she called me and told me that her doctor had informed her she was suffering from growing pains — the same as a seven year old child. Her muscles in her left side and along her spine were getting stronger. Her doctor found she was standing two inches taller.

She reports that her vision has improved so amazingly that she no longer uses her glasses except to read.

"Rebounding is far better than wheelchairing," she tells me.

Dorothy has shared this story with many personal friends and because of her, many of them enjoy better health through rebounding.

DRAGI MILOR
Glendale, California

A letter written to Harold Coates, Burbank, Cal

Dear Mr. Coates:

On behalf of the members of Hi-Noon Optimist Club of Glendale, I want to thank you and your lovely wife, Judy, for the very interesting and educational program you presented to us recently on the subject of trampolines and their effect on our health. Specifically, you brought along a rebounder for demonstration by Judy.

Your program stressed the fact that the rebounder could very markedly improve the health, in a way that other forms of exercise could not, and do it safely, especially for older people.

As a result, several of our Hi-Noon Optimist Club members bought one of your rebounders for individual home use.

I am quite pleased with the results of the use of the rebounder. My wife is 68 and has had a severe arthritic problem, as well as a heart problem, for many years. I am 67 (going on 19).

I believe the rebounder is helping my wife quite a bit. It is reducing the daily pain quite a bit, increasing the circulation and flexibility of muscles. For myself, I find that I am getting by with less sleep necessary per night and am feeling better all the time.

If we can get these marked results in only one week, what would daily use of the rebounder accomplish in improved health over a period of years?

I am recommending the rebounder to all my friends, and if you wish, you can show this letter to anyone who might be interested in buying a rebounder.

Best wishes
Sincerely,
Dragi Milor

DM/d

HARRIS NELSON

Hollywood, California

Harris Nelson, Hollywood, California, has constructed the following letter which he sends out to anyone and everyone. He thought our readers may want to carry through with this type of an idea also.

"Dear _____:

"Since you are a good worthy friend, I have some good news I'd like to pass along to you. It could affect your life tremendously as it has mine. Sounds like a lousy TV commercial, but it's the truth. If you're health conscious, you'll read every word of this!

"Last March, 1978, it seemed that my body was falling apart trying to keep up with the rigors of living. I had had two heart attacks, losing four younger brothers (almost losing a fifth) to this same scourge, and I wondered how soon it would be my turn.

"I tried all forms of exercise but I couldn't stay with it. I even biked six miles a night for five years faithfully. All I did was exercise my "rear" and then I found out I couldn't WALK! It hurt. I "squeaked" all over. The slightest incline was an effort. I put on a bold front but I could no longer hide the limp caused by an arthritic hip and a chronic cough that had badgered me for years. The zip and enthusiasm has gone. I was ready to give up. I began to withdraw more and more. This was very much **unlike** Harris Nelson, who was now approaching 70.

"Then it happened! Another good friend revealed a brand new concept of exercising that he was handling and I bought it over the phone, sight unseen. I was ready for anything. Little did I know I was buying a sleeping giant that would revolutionize the exercising industry in the midst of the greatest exercising revolution this country has ever known.

"Today, I'm handling this miracle health machine called a rebounder . . . a small round trampoline, 10 inches high and about 38 inches across. All you do is bounce on it, very easily at first (convalescents can sit on it), and it's astounding how it massages every organ in the body. The results have been fantastic.

"It has been declared the MOST EFFECTIVE AND EFFICIENT EXERCISER EVER DEVISED BY MAN and no doctor has ever come forth to refute that statement.

"The concept is new. Bouncing puts all the cells in the body under stress. In defense they fortify themselves drawing on protein, strengthening their walls. They become stronger and SO DO YOU. It's as simple as that! And it works!

NOW, you can jog indoors and avoid the perils of the street. Besides, jogging on a hard surface is very detrimental to the bone structure and skeletal system, as any doctor will tell you. Here's what it has done for me in less than four months, exercising five minutes twice a day. That's all you need to keep fit!"

"I need only six hours of sleep at night now, and no tossing as before — and I wake up refreshed. No more getting up nights. Stress and anxiety reduced 100%. Cough gone; arthritis gone. I can eat anything now, even before going to bed and not waking up dizzy and nauseated at four in the morning because of a heart problem. I've never enjoyed better regularity or elimination — it's perfect. **NO ANGINA PAINS!** I have renewed zip and vitality. I've lost eight pounds in the process and no dieting. All muscles are firmer — "pot" reduced 1½ inches. I can read music faster. My mind reacts quicker — and I'm sure it corrects disorders I'm not even aware of. Plus, plus, plus . . .

"All this, and why? Better circulation — stronger lung power and a stimulated lymphatic system (your toxic poison and waste disposal) — action and movement. Exercise! And, happy day, I can do it all while watching television! No special garb, no sweat!

"Every family should have one — every office, for increased efficiency . . . instead of a coffee break, bounce!

"The old folks love it, you can't keep the kids off of it and the dog finds it the coolest spot in town.

"AND, look at this: REBOUNDING REPLACES ALL OTHER EXERCISES. It's all you need and it's so delightfully fun. It's an exercise you'll be able to maintain and stay with it! Share it with the whole family.

"The cost is about equal to one day in a hospital. 'Tis better to spend it **now** to preclude that "visitation?!"

"I'd love to give you a demonstration with no obligation. Please call me.

"Yours for service and better health."

At the bottom of this letter, Harris wrote, "Why have a heart attack? Get the 'jump' on it!" I think this letter is GREAT!

WALT and DOROTHY ROSS

West Covina, Cal.

Walt and Dorothy Ross stopped by our office to say "Hello" while passing through on a trip recently. They are two beautiful people with a great testimony, so we asked them to write it down and send it to us. Here it is, just as we received it:

"Dear Al:

"Following is Walt's and my testimony of rebound exercise.

"DOROTHY ROSS — GRANDMOTHER OF TWENTY-ONE, and I feel as good as I did when I was THIRTY-FIVE but that wasn't true last February or years before.

"Early in the 1960's I was hospitalized for a pinched nerve and the X-Rays showed early arthritis had settled in the spine. Other illnesses came and the years were long with headaches, high blood pressure, ringing in the ears, and poor balance, arthritis spread to the right knee and both ankles, bursitis in the right shoulder and both hips, constant backache and always a feeling of complete exhaustion.

"This was the story of my life — I worked four mornings a week and I would drag myself out of bed, prepare for the day, fix breakfast and go to work. At noon I managed to prepare a lunch for myself and my husband Walt, get him off to work then go to bed, fighting to awake at four or five o'clock in the afternoon to prepare dinner and back to bed again, sometimes as early as seven or eight o'clock. I cried many a night from bursitis pain, so Walt bought a four inch foam pad to go over the mattress. Still the pain. Mind you, all of this going on for years on end, under constant doctor's care and being told that I was just getting old and had to expect this sort of thing.

"Walt was having his problems too. He suffered a heart attack while an aerospace executive, became a diabetic a few years ago, and had four cancer surgeries last year, two of them within twenty-eight days.

"We had tried various exercise programs. Bicycling

was impossible because of an arthritic knee, the door gyms were not effective, walking was not consistent, and it had been too many years for the barbells. All of this discouragement brought us to pray for some form of exercise or something that would help us to overcome our problems so we could enjoy our work and daily lives.

"Just a week after fervent prayer Walt was introduced to the rebounder. He bought the first unit that night and hurried home to show it to me and to exercise on it. He was excited. For three days I watched him do this thirty seconds at a time and each day he seemed brighter and had more energy. His disposition was bright and sunny and he literally began to whistle while he worked. Well, I thought this was all in his mind, because I just could not see how that simple exercise could make such a change in anyone in any length of time, much less in just three days!

"With his example I tried to use the rebounder, but could not keep my balance, so he held my hands to steady me and for three days, morning and evening I did twenty-five counts of the gentle health bounce and sure enough I, too, began to feel better. I, too, began to have more stamina and in two weeks my blood pressure dropped thirty points, I lost eight pounds and began to sing while I worked — literally! No more afternoons in bed; the rebounder replaced those three and four hour naps, and life took on a whole new outlook. I had felt so tired, had hurt for so long, and had headaches for days on end that I truly had forgotten how it felt to feel really GOOD — NO, REALLY GREAT!

"After two and a half months of proper exercise a metamorphosis had taken place. My backaches were gone, no more headaches, arthritis and bursitis pain, leg or foot cramps, and I lost twenty pounds and three dress sizes from a 24½ to a 18½. If that wasn't enough, I heal more quickly and sleep soundly for the first time in years. NO WONDER I FEEL AS GOOD AS I DID

WHEN I WAS THIRTY-FIVE!

"What has rebound exercise done for Walt?

"His stamina and recuperative powers have reached phenomenal dimensions. He has lost eighteen pounds and within a short period of time he could run a mile. His cholesterol level, which had always been high and was the cause of his heart attack, was ten points below normal. His heart beat has grown slow and steady, dropping eight beats per minute. His eye sight has cleared so that he now drives and watches television without glasses. He has been told by his doctor he could be free of diabetes completely in a few months. The doctor also stated that Walt is now in better physical condition than at any time since he has known him.

"We've had two vacation trips since starting the rebounder last spring, and we left other things home in order to take the rebounder with us. All along the way it was the first thing into the room. We exercised morning asnd night. We knew it would keep us feeling

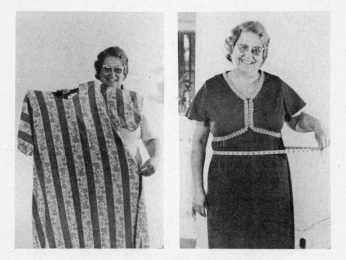

great and we enjoyed our trips so much more than we had in many years.

"Are we thrilled, excited and anxious to share the unbelievable benefits of the rebounder? We certainly are! Our whole life has changed for the better. We are happier, healthier, busier and more eager for each new day.

"Our enthusiasm was such that Walt became an administrator within thirty days and has been bringing health and happiness and prosperity to many others.

Sincerely,
Walt and Dorothy Ross
West Covina, CA

P.S. Both of Walt's doctors were so impressed with his rapid recovery and physical progress after using the rebounder that it took only fifteen seconds to convince them that each of them needed a unit in their own home! Isn't that exciting?!"

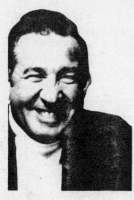

FRANK ANGELO
Akron, Penn.

Frank Angelo is a human dynamo of energy and enthusiasm. Ask him about health and he'll tell you. Don't ask him about health, and he'll still tell you.

Weighing 120 pounds and 5'1", he claims he is in better condition now than when he graduated from college as a physical education major, almost 30 years ago.

In 1970, Frank found himself standing in front of a mirror in his swimming suit, in a state of shock, disbelief and utter dispair. When he looked down he couldn't see his toes! He weighed 160 pounds and suddenly he couldn't stand the funny little fat man staring back at him. Something had to be done.

The next few years was the ole' diet routine. He lost and gained and lost, reaching a plateau 20 pounds lighter. His body was not trim, tanned, and tight as it used to be, but soft and flabby.

Around Christmas 1976, Frank was introduced to rebound exercise. Now, two years later, you'll find him bouncing (literally) all over the United States, enthusiastically telling all of his friends and their friends about rebound exercise. When asked why, Frank answers with a sparkle in his eye, "Well, I have just kept enjoying it. My body is very trim and firm at 120 pounds. I have energy galore. I sleep a lot less than I used to. I think more clearly and my entire life has taken on a new

157

bounce. I have dropped from 160 to 120 pounds. I am trying to share these facts with as many people as I can. There are millions of people like me who want to look better and feel better.''

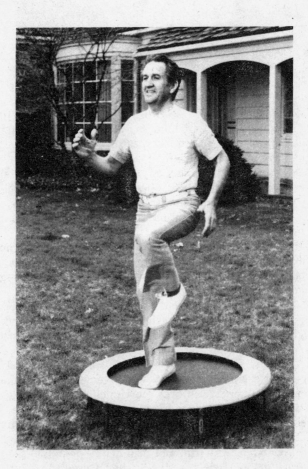

LAVERNE GROFF
Stevens, Pennsylvania

LaVern, 28, is sharing her story hoping it will help and encourage many people.

. . . "And they were married and lived happily ever after . . . Some fairy tales end that way. The first seven years of my married life was more of a nightmare because I was in and out of hospitals more times than I would like to remember. Less than a year after we were married, my husband rushed me to the hospital. After the operation, my doctor told me I was lucky to be alive. My ovary had ruptured and I had been bleeding internally. He had to remove half the ovary. Less than a year later the same thing happened to the other half — back to the hospital for the same operation. The third operation came when the other ovary ruptured less than nine months later. Each time I was admitted bigger tumors and cysts began appearing. As I was recovering from my third operation in the recovery room, my heart stopped! Quick action of the doctors and nurses started it beating again.

A week later, after various tests, my doctor informed me that they had found something else that had to be corrected. "Oh, not me. Not again. It just can't be," I cried. But it was.

With all of the operations and convalescence I was not able to exercise. A short time after my last operation, my body just gave up. My nerves and muscles no longer functioned. I practically became a vegetable. I couldn't talk for over two months. Someone had to feed me. I didn't have the strength to lift my arms. Walking was impossible. My back muscles were so weak that I was always in pain. I began seeing a chiropractor who really did help me a lot. As I began to learn to walk all over again I was in constant pain from my back and my operations.

"Oh, Lord, isn't there any hope?" I prayed.

My husband and I were introduced to rebound exercise by attending one of Dr. Corwin West's self-help clinics. He told me that he had seen only one person in a worse physical condition. We followed Dr. West's instructions. At first, I had to sit next to a rebounder with my feet on the mat while my husband bounced. We did this a few minutes several times a day. In a few weeks, I was on it myself — sitting at first — then standing. As months went by, I could feel my strength coming back. It was almost like climbing out of a grave into a flowery meadow. I was alive. And the pain was disappearing. Not only were my arms and legs getting stronger, I could also feel my insides get stronger. Both my family doctor and my chiropractor could not believe that I was the same person.

We will have had our rebounder one year the end of May and we wouldn't give it up for all the world. We also have the most wonderful news that could have ever happened to us. We are now expecting our first baby the end of August. The doctor said that if I hadn't received so much strength to my insides, I could never be carrying this baby. Considering the fact that we did it with only half an ovary, we thank our dear Lord each day for leading us to Dr. West, Frank and Cathy Angelo, and the rebounder.

I would like everyone to know this rebounder is the best thing I have ever found for eliminating pain without pills.

I am now up to 15 minutes of running and jumping on the rebounder at a time several times a day and I feel just wonderful!"

LaVern Groff gave birth to a six pound baby. Naturally, the doctors expected complications, but after keeping the baby in the hospital for five weeks, they found the baby perfectly normal and healthy. Mother and baby are now happy and healthy and, of course, dad struts like a proud peacock!

BLAKE STEEL, 33
Eugene, Oregon

Blake is working full time selling storm windows in Eugene, Oregon. That doesn't seem unusual until you learn that he has suffered most of his life from a birth defect in his lower back which caused his spine to torque or twist, causing constant tension and cramping in his back and neck, keeping him always in pain.

At 30, he made the decision to have his back fused to relieve the pain. The surgery involved taking bone from his hip and fusing the lower vertebrae to the sacrum. After surgery, from May to January, Blake could not do anything because of the pain every time he moved. He was weaker than before. Eight months after surgery an X-ray revealed that the fusion did not take. His doctor informed him that his only hope was an other fusion. This time they would open him up through his abdomen and fuse the front of his spine. There had to be another way.

It was at this time that he was introduced to rebound exercise. He started slowly because of the pain and his weakened muscle condition.

Through constant use of the rebounder every day, though many times he was in pain, his muscles began to respond and strengthen. After 6 months of exercise the pain diminished. The tension and cramping of his back and neck have been eliminated as long as he rebounds every day. After living with constant pain for 13 years, it's easy to see why he is so enthused about rebound exercise — especially since he did not need the second operation.

Blake is working full time — and is feeling better at 33 than he did when he was a teenager.

"Consistancy is the most important thing," says Blake, when asked what advice he would like to give others who are considering rebounding for exercise.

NORMAN NIELSON
Edmonds, Washington

On July 13th 1960 Norm's life changed drastically. Nielson, 38, was pulled out of his crumpled automobile and rushed to the hospital where he remained in a semi-conscious condition for over 75 days with a crushed spine. He was released from hospital in October and wheeled home to convalesce. Determined not to let a small accident get in his way Norm began his long climb out of his wheel chair through constant exercise and will power.

February 1961 he went to work, walking — slowly, but walking. His recovery was so remarkable that in 1963 he began driving an Econoline Van for his company, covering Oregon and Washington. Things were looking good for Norm and his family until sometime in 1965 when he began dragging his right foot. He began to notice numbness in his leg and entire right side. It was finally decided that his doctor should perform an exploratory laminectomy to find the cause of the increasing lack of control. The back half of a number of vertebrae in the middle of his back were removed to reveal that the nerves in his spinal chord was filling with scar tissue. His wound was closed and he was informed that he would gradually become numb from his feet to the top of the injury which was about the middle of his chest. By 1967 he was working from a wheel chair and in 1968 he was released from work on an early disability retirement.

IN 1970 Norm was admitted to 6th North at the University of Washington to learn how to be self sufficient as a paraplegic. He had to learn how to exercise with pulleys, while his patient, loving wife faithfully helped put his body through its full range of motion every morning before she went to work.

The muscles in his legs and his buttocks atrophied until there was very little flesh between his skin and

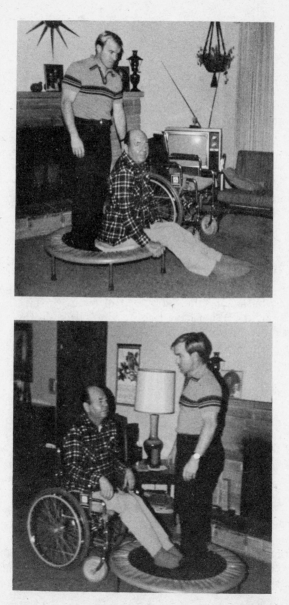

bones. He had to sit on special pillows to keep from getting bed sores.

Losing control of his excretory capabilities made matters even worse. Every day became a strict regimen of timing and exercise just to be able to survive.

The next eight years seemed a slow descent to deeper troubles. Finally, Norm found that it was impossible for ¼ of his body to lift the other ¾ of his virtually dead body. If he fell out of his wheel chair he had to call his wife home from work to help him get back in.

Norm became concerned about the lack of circulation in his legs. A friend of his in similar circumstances, lost by surgery first his toes, then his foot. The third operation took his leg from the knee down. He did not want to go through this dehumanizing and expensive experience.

About the middle of August, 1978 Norm was introduced to rebound exercise. After a brief explanation of the basic concepts, he agreed to try it. "After all," he thought, "What have I got to lose?" His wheel chair was rolled up to the rebounder and his numb feet and legs were placed in the middle of the rebounder for about five minutes. Next, Norm was lifted out of his wheelchair and placed on his special pillow sitting in the middle of the rebounder. With someone standing behind him, providing the bounce, Norm began his new way of life.

At this writing, Norm Nielson has been rebounding at least five days a week for the last four months at least one hour a day, a half hour sitting in his wheelchair next to the rebounder with his feet in the middle, and another half hour sitting on the rebounder.

The High Priests Group of the Edmonds First Ward of the Church of Jesus Christ of Latter Day Saints has made certain that someone was there every day volunteering their time to help him in and out of his chair. His neighbors have also made sure someone was there to assist him.

The following are changes that have been noticed by Norm, his family and friends.

1. Within the first three days skin tone color was seen in his right foot instead of steel gray.
2. 100% improvement in lung capacity within first week.
3. Healthier flesh tone color to the entire right side of his body, especially to his face.
4. Increasing feeling sensations to the lower three-fourths of his body that had been numb for 11 years.
5. he is able to separate his knees by the use of his muscles — something he hasn't been able to do for nine years.
6. Norm has noticed feelings in the muscles in his back, just above his belt for the first time in 11 years.
7. He has also noticed that his legs have become more fleshy and some muscle in his buttocks has developed where before there was nothing.
8. He has more energy making it possible to stay awake longer making a longer day without feeling tired all day long.
9. He has stronger arms and upper body making it easier to transfer higher and further.
10. He has changed from a 14½" shirt collar to a 16" shirt collar.
11. He is much warmer during the day — no longer needs a sweater.
12. Norm claims his elimination has improved 1000%! (We who do not have that problem do not know what he is talking about.)
13. His lovely wife says that he is easier to get along with.
14. According to the University of Washington, at his last physical checkup he reduced his blood pressure from 152/95 to 124/80.

15. Norm feels it is important to note that although the energy necessary for him to rebound comes from external means by other people assisting him by providing the bounce, he has noticed he has reduced his waistline and tightened his stomach.

Norm Nielson is no longer dead from the chest down. He is very much alive. We don't know what the future will bring, but if the last four months are any indication, he is in for a long steady climb. He is pleased with his progress and is willing to wait. It is we who are healthy who always seem to be impatient.

PAT GLASPIE

My name is Pat Glaspie and I reside in Ritzville, Washington. I was born with cerebral palsy which affected my right side. Two years ago, I was introduced to rebound exercise. After eleven days on a rebounder, I was able to wiggle two of my right toes. I was so thrilled I became very dedicated to exercising on the rebounder very faithfully. My health wasn't at all good at that time plus the fact that I was thirty pounds overweight.

Within two months, I lost 27 pounds and went from a size 16 to a size 10, and in three month's time, I was able to control my entire right foot. I now have control over my complete right side!

As if cerebral palsy was not affliction enough, I also had hypoglycemia and spent at least seven days each month in bed from pure exhaustion because this disease caused my heart to beat as high as 200 beats per minute. This also put me in a very despondent mood most of the time, and at times I was sure I would die before the day was over. Through much study of rebound exercise, I knew the rebounder would help this problem also.

About this same time, I attended lectures given by Dr.

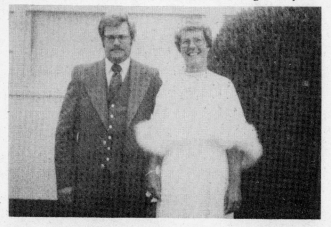

C. Samuel West, D.N., to learn how to eliminate poisons from the body. Between rebound exercise and Dr. West, the hypoglycemia was completely gone from my body within seven months.

I became so sold on rebounders that I had to let the rest of the world know my new-found exercise, so I began lecturing to small groups and selling rebounders.

I now lecture all over the eastern part of Washington. I like to think I am a combination of Al Carter and Dr. West. I teach diet, lymphatics and rebound exercise and today I thank the Lord that I am a new woman with a bright future of good health and financial success! What more could anyone ask?

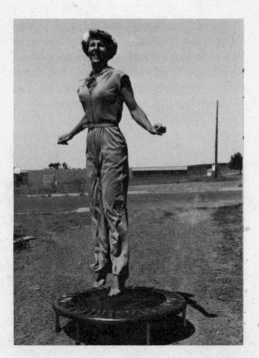

STEVE WORTHINGTON

Salt Lake City, Utah

My name is Steve Worthington and I reside in Salt Lake City, Utah. In January, 1978, I entered the hospital to have a disc removed from my back which had been bothering me for seven or eight years. Before I had this operation, the doctor informed me I would be out of work approximately five to six months.

On January 9, 1978, surgery was performed and the L-4 disc in my back was removed. Two days later, the doctors came in, had me out of the bed, standing and walking around. On January 15, I was released from the hospital and sent home. The doctors told me to just lay around and take it easy and do a minimal amount of walking.

On January 30, 1978, Brent Hermanson, an administrator in the Trim Way Distributors Association, introduced me to rebound exercising. I purchased a unit at that time and started out just walking gradually on the unit for maybe five to ten minutes a day. I did this for the first week and then I increased the activity by jogging, twisting and jumping lightly on the rebounder.

I continued to do this until February 25, when I had to go back to the doctor for an appointment to be re-examined and to check on my progress. At that time, the doctor informed me I had made a remarkable recovery from the surgery. He had me do various exercises in his office to check on my mobility and stability, etc. He said he saw no reason why I shouldn't be able to return to work. He released me to go back to my position as a railroad engineer, effective March 1, 1978.

January 2, 1978, I weighed 260 pounds. I didn't feel I was in very good health and was determined I was going to lose weight and become physically fit. While I was in the hospital, I limited my amount of food and started on a diet to lose weight. By the time I was introduced to the rebounder, I had lost probably ten pounds. Since that time up to this present date, I have lost over thirty pounds. I contribute most of that to spending twenty-five minutes a day doing rebound exercises. I now feel in better shape than I have ever been in the past fifteen years. The rebounder is certainly the way to go and maintain and keep a vigorous, healthy life!

GEORGE JANSON   Tiffin, Ohio

George Janson, 58, is the Athletic Director of Tiffin University and because it is a small institution he is also the basketball coach. George was introduced to rebounding as an exercise about a year ago by Charles Boice of Modesto, California. It took very little to convince George that rebounding was a valuable way to exercise especially for himself. But because it was new he wanted to see if it would also help his basketball team.

After 60 days of home rebounding, although he had been playing less golf, his game improved and was verified by his golf pro. His score dropped from around 100 to the low 80's! Naturally, both George and his golf pro were amazed. "I feel it's the overall body coordination that one achieves through rebounding," says George. "but wait till you hear what our basketball team has done with the rebounder."

Mr. Janson usually has the rebounder on the side of the basketball floor for immediate warm up for the player called into the game. He claims three reasons for using the rebounder during a game: "First it psychs up our player; second, it psychs out our opponent; and, third, it really works!"

The rebounder is used during practice to improve their vertical jumps to the basket.

"Any basketball coach will tell you that vertical jumping practice beyond a minute and a half will drain a good player. That's why they usually put it at the end of practice. We use the rebounder under the basket and after three minutes it not only improves the basketball rebounding but they feel rejuvenated and ready to play.

"Those are the vital statistics of one of your young athletes," his doctor exclaimed, as he verified Janson's blood pressure at 120/80 and pulse of 68. "What are you doing?"

George explained and his doctor bought a rebounder.

MICHAEL J. FRANK
(The son of James B. Frank)

Tiffin, Ohio

Mike purchased a rebounder for his father who just 30 days earlier was released from the Cleveland Clinic to recuperate from open heart surgery. Controlled exercise was vitally important to James B. Frank. Here are some excerpts from his report from the Cleveland Clinic.

October 24, 1978
425 Clinton Ave.
Tiffin, Ohio 44883

Dear Al:

Enclosed please find the results of my blood tests and the picture of my father and myself which you asked me to send to you.

You can see the incredible decline in the level of Triglycerides in just two months. After the first test, the doctor placed me on a 1500-2000 calorie diet and told me to get plenty of exercise.

I purchased my rebounder at the end of June, 1978. It was only after I began my rebound exercises, that I experienced the weight loss which contributed a great deal to the decrease in my lipid profile. I went from 160¼ to 152 lbs. in just one month.

As I briefly explained to you, the main reason I purchased a rebounder was not for myself, but for my father. His story is far more "miraculous" than mine. I will quote you some excerpts from the final report from the Cleveland Clinic. RE: Mr. James B. Frank.

"On February 27, 1978 he suffered an acute and extensive anteroseptal myocardial infarction which awakened him from sleep. He was hospitalized at Mercy Hospital in Tiffin, Ohio, and suffered from transient complete heart block and a pacemaker was implanted temporarily.

After 21 days he was discharged from the hospital, but a week later he slipped into pulmonary edema and was readmitted with intractable congestive heart failure. His chest film was quite alarming and showed a bulge on the left heart border due to a ventricular aneurysm. His congestion was severe and he was transferred to the Cleveland Clinic for further treatment on April 2, 1978.

Upon admission to the Clinic he was in acute distress with congestive heart failure. The chest x-ray showed cardiac enlargement, ventricular aneurysm, and pulmonary congestion.

He experienced some premature heart beats and a short run of ventricular tachycardia. To combat this he was started on a relatively new drug — Norpace.

However, he vomited the doses of Norpace and during this period of time he suffered a cardiac arrest. Luckily, his wife was present and several medical residents were able to resuscitate him with no neurological deficit. He was then transferred to the Intensive Care Unit.

He was stabilized for one week so as to allow the scar tissue around the infarction to firm up in order to perform a ventricular aneurysm resection. Ideally, elective aneurysmectomy is carried out three months after an infarction, but in this case we were unable to wait that long. His heart failure and ventricular arrhythmias dictated earlier surgery.

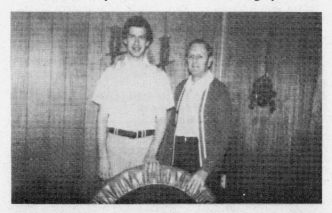

Mr. Frank underwent open heart surgery on April 17, 1978. A segment measuring 10 cm. x 6 cm. was removed with a good sized adherent mural thrombus as well. His recovery was a little slow but steady. He was discharged in good condition on May 3, 1978."

As I'm sure you can see from this report, my father is indeed fortunate to still be alive. He is feeling quite well, all things considered, and has resumed working on a full-time basis.

Both my father and myself want to thank you very much for taking the time to come to Tiffin. Your lecture provided us with both needed information and example to enable us to develop our rebound exercise programs.

You have certainly sold us on the value of rebound exercise and you can be sure that we will promote the value of the rebounder to our friends and neighbors.

Mr. Frank has been rebuilding the strength of his body with the use of the Rebounder a few minutes each day because it is easy and convenient. He feels he has complete control of the surrounding environment. Jim Frank is now back to work on a full time basis.

Although Mike secured the Rebounder for his father, Mike began using it also. A recent medical examination by his own doctor, Robert R. Pagarigan, M.D. of Tiffin, dictated that he too should be concerned about his own health habits.

ANTHONY S. LUPICA, M.D.
ROBERTO R. PAGARIGAN, M.D.
40 CLAY STREET
TIFFIN, OHIO 44883

October 23, 1978
RE: Mike Frank

TO WHOM IT MAY CONCERN:

The above named patient had the following test drawn on May 25th 1978 Lipid 720 mg. percent
  Cholesterol 220 mg.
  Triglycerides 205 mg. percent— (33-185)

July 28th, 1978 Lipid 640 mg percent
  Cholesterol 190 mg percent
  Triglycerides 105 mg percent

ANTHONY S. LUPICA, M.D.

JIM VOLK
Twin Falls, Idaho

Rebound Exercise may be in the next issue of the Guinness Book of World Records.

Jim Volk, 36, of Twin Falls, Idaho, did 16,062 jumping jack exercises in three hours and 43½ minutes eclipsing the officially listed World Record by 2½ minutes. He then went on to do 18,300 jumps in four hours 18 minutes and 23 seconds. He did it on a rebounder!

"I think doing this number of exercises proves that rebounding eliminates most of the shock to the system. A couple of years ago when I attempted to break the record, I had to stop at 12,000 because my legs were sore and numb from the knees down. My arms and shoulders were so sore that I wasn't able to raise my arms another time," said Volk.

"I felt good throughout the whole time this time. I started at 80 per minute, averaged 75 the first hour and slowed only to one jumping jack a second in the final few minutes."

When asked why he stopped, Volk stated "I just felt that 2,000 over the World Record was enough and I had to stop sometime."

"How did he feel afterwards?"

"There was just a little bit of soreness in the ankles and shoulders. I wasn't at all tired but instead felt more alert and alive afterwards. It definitely does provide a positive effect on the system."

"After 3 hours of running on a hard surface, my legs would feel heavy. Now I run in place on the rebounder and strengthen the muscles without the 'bone jarring' shock."

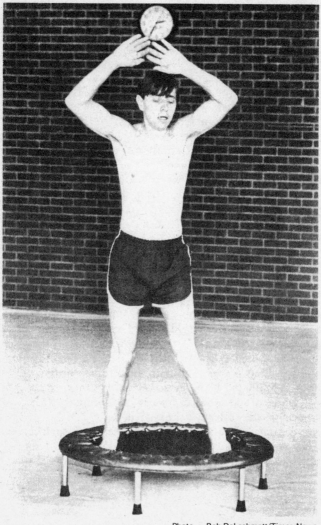

Photo — Bob DeLashmatt/Times-News
Twin Falls, Idaho

176

LORI CALL

Edmonds, Washington

For the past 25 years I have suffered with the excruciating pain of bursitis in my right elbow and shoulder. I have had the usual medical treatments to include ultra sonic sound without any lasting relief or improvement. In addition, for the past 3 years I have had severe pain in my knees, making it impossible to sit in one place for any length of time. When it was first suggested to me that rebound exercise would take away my pain, I simply scoffed at the idea. I was smart enough to know that bouncing up and down would not help a condition I had suffered with for years. It took some persuasion but I finally tried the rebounder, knowing full well I was wasting my time.

I wasn't very diligent at first and had to be reminded to use the rebounder. To my surprise and delight in about two weeks I began to notice that the pain in my elbow and shoulder was improving. For the next two weeks I was careful to use the rebounder every day. By the end of the next two weeks I was functioning without pain in either my knees, elbow or shoulder. During the holidays I slacked off and within two weeks I noticed the pain in my knees returning. Needless to say rebound exercise is and will continue to be a definite part of every day.

G.N. Getman, O.D.
Chula Vista, California

Rebound tumbling is an activity that has enjoyed great popularity in the past few years. The Trampoline — the device for rebound tumbling — has usually been considered as gymnastic equipment, and too frequently one of its real values has been overlooked. The concern over the dangers of rebound tumbling has been exaggerated. When a few simple rules of caution and guidance are utilized, the Trampoline is less dangerous than many of the activities common to children.

The Trampoline provides opportunities for the acquisition of basic movement control, which is essential to coordination. Clinical and research studies of rebound tumbling indicate that the Trampoline can provide experiences that influence a child's academic success. Many authorities recognize that a child's freedom to learn and his readiness for new learning experiences is dependent upon his freedom and control of movement. This control of movement must come from the visual mechanism because eyes are the primary steering machinery for all movements.

The human being should be bilateral for freedom in movement. His success in movement and the development of coordination develop from his organization and the combination of his two halves. The bilaterality of the two body halves should be matched by the bilaterality of the two eyes. This teaming of body and eyes allows a child to come to a functional and interpretive balance on every learning task.

The Trampoline contributes more to the organization of bilaterality than any other known device. On this basis, the following routines are recommended for all children, but especially for those whose lack of coordination and general clumsiness is evident in many areas of performance. Such clumsiness is most evident in many areas of performance. Such clumsiness is most evident to the optometrist who concerns himself with the visual efficiency that children need for success in academic tasks. These optometrists are recommending rebound tumbling for the improvements in **total** visual and body control. It is **not used** solely for building muscle bulk and strength.

— From Supplement to *Optometric Child Care & Guidance*

VISION THERAPY

by Dr. Theodore S. Kadet, O.D.
Issaquah, Washington

Developmental optometry, a specialty within the profession of optometry, has made effective use of rebounding for many years. We have found the rebounder to be a valuable tool for creating an awareness of using vision as the primary guiding system for movement. The inability to use vision efficiently as the major sensory system to the brain can be a primary cause of learning disabilities in children and adults. Our treatment of these visual perception dysfunctions is called vision therapy.

To better understand the role of rebounding in vision therapy, a brief background summary is helpful. Many parents of learning disabled children, suspecting vision problems, have consulted optometry for help and guidance. Symptoms such as letter and number reversals, awkward posture and handwriting, holding books very close to the eyes when reading, immaturity in physical and coordination development, and short visual attention span are reported by the parents.

Often, the standard vision analysis, which measures the optical components of each eye, eye balance and efficiency of the eyes to team together, provided little insight into the problem. Reporting this to the parents gave them little satisfaction and set us to wondering why such obvious vision problems were not being diagnosed by our routine examinations.

Research, spearheaded by such notables as A. M. Skeffington, O.D., G. N. Gettman, O.D., and D. B. Harmon, Ph.D., under the auspices of the Optometric Extension Program, provided some clues to answering our dilemma. The visual difficulties appeared to be inadequate visual perception development, usually along with immaturity of the other sensory systems.

We are born with the physical equipment for vision, audition, kinesthesis (movement), touch taste and smell.

However, we **learn** to use these systems to gather information about our environment. This learning, or maturing, begins in infancy and continues throughout our lifetime. Taste and smell mature most quickly in infancy, followed by movement and touch which begin maturing rapidly at six months to one year. The vision and auditory systems mature more slowly, reaching rapid development at 18 months to two years of age. The Gesell Institute of Child Development in New Haven, Connecticut, has done mammoth research into human growth and development, providing much of our knowledge in this area.

In some children, sensory development of all systems appears to take place at a slower rate of speed. This may be due to inadequate environmental stimulation by the parents, physical handicaps, neurological impairment, or just a slow "time clock." When ready to begin school at age five or six, these children are unable to use the vision and auditory systems as effective learning tools. Many of these children are still using the movement and touch systems as primary learning modes. Unfortunately, movement and touch skills are not of much value in a classroom environment.

In vision therapy, we attempt to help "Mother Nature" along in the development of the vision and vision-auditory interaction systems by creating an environment where these systems will mature at a more rapid rate. We concentrate in such areas as visually guided body movements; visual size, space, form and direction relationships; visual-auditory integration; figure-ground relationships; visualization and visual memory skills. These skill areas provide the tools with which a child learns to read and do other school skills. As the skill level in these key areas improves, school performance often shows a corresponding improvement.

The rebounder is used to bring about efficient visually guided movement of the entire body. Rebounding gives magnificent feedback as to what the child did, thus bringing about a rapid awareness of using vision to guide movement. The rebounder is often used to bring about directional awareness, especially right and left. Confusion in this area often results in letter and word reversals.

Some developmental optometrists use the rebounder in working with athletes to develop better concentration when participating in their individual sports. Many professional teams have developmental optometrists working with their players to help them perform more accurately and efficiently.

In summary, the rebounder has found a welcome home in offices of developmental optometrists. We are very aware of the additional benefits rebounding provides as a secondary impact to the areas of our concern. All professions dealing with people are becoming more aware of the need to treat the entire person, not just part of him. Developmental optometry watches with great interest developments in all fields which contribute to allowing every person to reach his highest potential.

GIDEON ARIEL, PH.D.
Director, Computerized Biomedical Analysis

Amherst, Massachusetts

Dr. Gideon Ariel, founder of Computerized Biomechanical Analysis, Inc., is an internationally known expert in the field of biomechanics. His own experience as an Olympic athlete representing Israel in 1960 and 1964, combined with the acquisition of a Ph.D. in both exercise science and computer science, laid the groundwork for his current research into the mechanics of human motion. Dr. Ariel is responsible for revolutionary changes in the scientific design and testing of sports equipment — a field in which he is recognized as a pioneer.

Conducting research for such prestigious corporations as A.M.F., Spalding and Universal Gym, Dr. Ariel has eliminated some of the guesswork, previously unavoidable in product design, through his innovative use of computer science. The dramatic results hae been felt by manufacturers and consumers, as well as by victims of muscular dystrophy and other motor-related deficiencies.

Dr. Ariel is presently involved in the writing of a book which details practical applications of his scientific findings.

THE EFFECT OF DIFFERENT PRACTICE REGIMENS ON ACCURACY OF THE TENNIS FOREHAND STROKE

The ability of the tennis player to accurately place the ball in specific court locations is an important component of tennis. A number of factors influence the ability of the player in accomplishing this goal including the body position of the player at the time of racquetball impact, the distance between the player and the ball, the speed of the ball, and the distance of the player from the target. In order to improve the player's ability in placing his shots in the desired locations, various training routines may be tried. For example, merely practicing the game itself usually promotes improvement. In addition, utilization of drills with throwing machines or repetitive hitting against a rebound wall may improve the placing ability.

The purpose of the present study was to test the effect of practicing the forehand while bouncing on a miniature trampoline. It was hypothesized that constant adjustment of the body to overcome the "moving ground" effect would *stimulate neuromuscular centers* thus producing greater ball placement skills.

METHOD

Six subjects, each with a minimum of 5 years exerience, were used in the present study. Their height varied between 165 and 187 cm. and their weight between 61 and 86 kg. The subjects were divided equally into control and experimental groups. A plywood board 4 feet by 8 feet with a 30 inch diameter hole in the center was used as the target. A throwing machine delivered the tennis ball at 35 mph to a location on the ground so that the ball bounced to approximately the hip height of the subject.

The frequency of ball delivery was one ball every five seconds. The players were instructed to use the forehand in attempting to hit the ball into the hole in the target board. The subject scored one point for each ball hit into the hole on the target board. Subjects attended 3 sessions each week with 100 practice hits per session. The control group practiced the forehand while standing on the floor. The experimental group practiced while bouncing on the miniature trampoline. Two evaluations were made of the practice tests.

Prior to the initial testing session all subjects were assessed in the number of points scored while standing on the floor. The location of the test was the same as that used by the control group in their practice sessions. The subjects were retested following the twenty-fifth practice session. A second evaluation compared the scores of the two groups, that is, the scores obtained while bouncing with those resulting from standing on the floor. All data were statistically analyzed.

RESULTS

Table 1 illustrates the results for the experimental and control groups performed on ground and on the miniature trampoline. The individual scores and the mean results are reported for each group. It was revealed that accuracy in hitting the target increased significantly for both groups. However, when measuring both groups on the ground, the experimental group achieved significantly greater results.

Table 2 illustrates the experimental results for the pre and post training sessions for both groups when measured standing on the floor. When tested under the same condition, the control group increased their performance by 13.34 percent while the experimental group improved 30.33 percent.

TABLE 1

EXPERIMENTAL RESULTS FOR EXPERIMENTAL AND CONTROL GROUPS PERFORMED ON GROUND AND THE REBOUND EXERCISE UNIT

	CONTROL		EXPERIMENTAL
	16 14 11	PERCENT INCREASE	15 9 10
MEAN:	13.67		11.33

TABLE 2

EXPERIMENTAL RESULTS FOR PRE AND POST TRAINING FOR BOTH GROUPS TESTED ON GROUND

	PRE-TRAINING	POST-TRAINING
	CONTROL GROUP	
	17	28
	15	30
	20	34
MEAN:	17.3	30.67
	DIFF% 13.34	
	EXPERIMENTAL GROUP	
	USING REBOUND EXERCISE	
	14	38
	15	47
	16	51
MEAN:	15.0	45.33
	DIFF% 30.33	

MEANS DIFFERENCES   17.0%
F-Ratio   12.02 (1,4)*
              Significant to the .05 level of confidence.

Dr. Ariel concludes that testing results show, — a player using rebound exercise as a tennis teaching aid in practice drills improves his accuracy efficiency more than 100% over a player going through the same practice drill and repetitions, but who does not use a rebounder as an aid.

DISCUSSIONS AND CONCLUSIONS

The present experiment illustrates that using the elusive, *it appears that certain modalities contribute to neuromuscular adjustment facilitating motor ability. For some yet unexplained reason, practicing the forehand while bouncing on the trampoline facilitates neuromuscular patterns, control signals, coordination, etc. resulting in increased accuracy.*

As with all scientific findings, additional research should examine a larger sample, other tennis strokes, different ball speeds and distance from the target. HOWEVER, "it would appear, that tennis players can improve both motor ability and, undoubtedly, general fitness by practicing tennis strokes while bouncing on a rebound exercise unit."

Bibliography

1 *"The New Book of Knowledge."* Encyclopedia Grolier, Inc. 1974 p. 320.

2 Brachet, J. *"The Cell"* Volume I, New York, Academic Press 1970.

3 *Doctrine & Covenants* 130:20-21 pub. Church of Jesus Christ of Latter-Day Saints, 1978.

4 *Physiology of Exercise* Morehouse, L.E. Ph.D. & Miller, A.J. Jr., Ph.D., M.D., The C.V. Mosby Co. 1969. p. 52.

5 *Ibid. p. 47*

6 *Human Anatomy and Physiology,* King, B., Ph.D. & Showers, M.J., Ph.D., The W.B. Sanders Co., 1963. p. 114.

7 *Bibliography of Space Medicine.* National Library of Medicine, Reference Division, Washington, 1968. and *U.S. Armed Forces Medical Journal,* 1969.

8 *Medical Physiology,* Guyton, A.C., M.D., W.B. Saunders Co., 1962. p. 31.

9 *Ibid. p. 65.*

10 *Ibid. p. 73.*

11 *Ibid. p. 4.*

12 *Ibid.* Chapter 2.

13 *Human Anatomy,* Schaeffer, J.P. (editor). McGraw-Hill, Inc. 1963. p. 399.

14 Medical Physiology. Guyton, A.C., M.D., W.B. Saunders Co. Chapter 4.

15 "Once-Frustrated Fitness Fiends are Jumping for Joy" C. Colgan article, *World-Wide Report* Feb. 1978. p. 12.

16 "But! Johnny Can Read" article, *College of Optometrists in Vision Development,* 1971.

17 "Vision Therapy" L. Dusky, article *Town & Country Magazine,* March 1975.

18 *Do You Really Need Glasses,* Rosanes-Berrett, M.B., *Popular Library,* 1974.

19 "Vision Therapy" L. Dusky article, *Town & Country Magazine, March, 1975.*

20 *Do You Really Need Glasses,* Rosanes-Barrett, M.B., Popular Library, 1974.

It was only a month previous to the publishing of this book that several advocates of rebound exercise were sharing their experiences and teaching techniques. The comment was made by one, "We have learned so much in the last two years about rebound exercise. There should be an organized, ongoing investigation of benefits to the human body."

This recommendation has been heard. The National Institute of Reboundology and Health, Inc., has been formed for that purpose. Doctors, psychiatrists, visual specialists, health enthusiasts and mom and dad want and need statistical and clinical data to properly form professional opinions. We have begun probably the most exciting adventure in physical fitness at the most appropriate time since we are in the beginning of the largest physical fitness revolution the world has ever seen. The information developed by this study will eventually touch more lives than any other known exercise concept.

NOTES